I0699906

Psychiatric Aspects of Cancer

Advances in Psychosomatic Medicine

Vol. 18

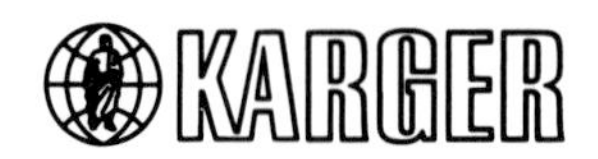

Basel · München · Paris · London · New York · New Delhi · Singapore · Tokyo · Sydney

Psychiatric Aspects of Cancer

Volume Editor
Richard J. Goldberg, Providence, R.I.
Psychiatrist-in-Chief, Rhode Island Hospital, Women and Infants Hospital;
Associate Professor, Departments of Psychiatry and Medicine, Brown University

4 tables, 1988

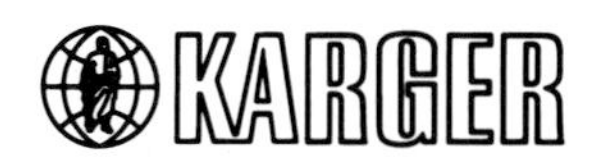

Basel · München · Paris · London · New York · New Delhi · Singapore · Tokyo · Sydney

Advances in Psychosomatic Medicine

Library of Congress Cataloging-in-Publication Data
Psychiatric aspects of cancer.
(Advances in psychosomatic medicine; vol. 18)
Includes bibliographies and index.
1. Cancer-Psychological aspects. I. Goldberg, Richard J., 1949-. II. Series. [DNLM: 1. Neoplasms-psychology. W1 AD81 v. 18/ QZ 200 P9723
RC262.P76 1988 616.99'4'0019 88-9286
ISBN 3-8055-4745-5

Bibliographic Indices
This publication is listed in bibliographic services, including Current Contents® and Index Medicus.

Drug Dosage

The authors and the publisher have exerted every effort to ensure that drug selection and dosage set forth in this text are in accord with current recommendations and practice at the time of publication. However, in view of ongoing research, changes in government regulations, and the constant flow of information relating to drug therapy and drug reactions, the reader is urged to check the package insert for each drug for any change in indications and dosage and for added warnings and precautions. This is particularly important when the recommended agent is a new and/or infrequently employed drug.

ISBN 3-8055-4745-5

Contents

Foreword

A potential reader of this volume is interested, undoubtedly, in the comprehensive clinical management of cancer patients. It is unfortunate that clinicians working in cancer care tend to be trained in a single discipline, since the impact of cancer and its treatment involves the patient and family in multiple interacting dimensions. In fact, the caregiver needs to try to encompass a variety of somatic and psychological domains, as well as the interaction between the physical and psychological — the psychosomatic. This book, as part of a series of *Advances in Psychosomatic Medicine*, does not address the 'psychosomatic' aspects of cancer from the viewpoint of cancer as a physical consequence of psychological processes. Instead, its 'psychosomatic' perspective addresses critical 'psychiatric', 'psychosocial' and 'somatic' aspects of cancer and their interactions. It is assumed that the reader has a background that tends to be stronger in either the psychosocial or the biological dimensions of cancer care. However, patients do not come so neatly packaged. It is hoped that this volume will provide important information basic to a 'psychosomatic' understanding and management of the cancer patient.

The *somatic* components of the 'psychosomatic' equation are represented in this volume by three chapters which contain information often appreciated best only by medically oriented psychiatrists working in this area. The evaluation of symptoms of distress cannot be limited to psychosocial factors alone. Nonmedically oriented clinicians need to become familiar with the possible medical factors underlying disturbed mood, thought or behavior and consider appropriate somatic treatments, including psychotropic medications. This psychiatric approach is reviewed by Drs. Massie and Holland in relation to depression. Among the 'psychosomatic' issues involving cancer patients is the question of the effects of cancer therapies on the central nervous system — an area covered in this volume by Drs. Silberfarb and Oxman. Finally, the recognition of delirium is critically important for cancer caregivers, especially since delirium often masquerades as a variety of psychosocial disturbances. Dr. Adams reviews issues pertinent to the recognition, diagnosis, and management of delirium in the many forms it takes in cancer patients.

The *psychological* dimensions of cancer are represented by three chapters. Dr. Wool addresses the issue of denial in cancer patients, a topic which touches upon every phase of the illness from its recognition to choices about treatment. Two modalities of psychological therapies are also represented. Dr. Linn reviews the *psychotherapies* as they apply to cancer patients. This chapter, like the others in this volume, is meant to be of practical clinical value, built upon a foundation of academically derived data. Drs. Spirito, Hewett, and Stark address a *behavioral therapy* approach to cancer-related clinical problems, to provide clinicians with a sense of what this dimension has to offer patients.

Finally, the *psychosocial* components of the 'psychosomatic' equation are represented by four contributions. Cancer does not take place in a vacuum. Its impact is felt by the family in ways that are reviewed by Dr. Northouse. Further, the availability, access to, and provision of 'concrete services' is a dimension of cancer care which interacts in powerful ways with the psychological and somatic course of the illness. No matter what the orientation of the caregiver, a broader understanding of and support for development of adequate services for the patient is necessary. The role of concrete services is reviewed by Drs. Mor, Guadagnoli, and Wool. In addition, the Hospice Model of Care is included and reviewed by Dr. Mor and Ms. Masterson-Allen because this model of care serves as a paradigm for provision of services using a 'psychosomatic' approach, which attempts to integrate the psychological and concrete service needs with the necesssary medical aspects of therapy. Finally, Dr. Slaby addresses the impact of cancer care on the providers. Much has been written about the stress of providing care to cancer patients and the incidence of professional burn-out which results. Reflection on the providers' issues may prompt the reader to seek a broader conceptual framework as the basis for the care of cancer patients.

This volume hopes to place various psychologic and somatic components of cancer care in a broader conceptual framework. Providers cannot afford for themselves or for the sake of their patients to cling exclusively to a unidimensional approach to the distressed patient. By learning to encompass the relevance of dimensions usually relegated to other professions, each provider will become more effective in helping to create a more rational and effective system of care for the cancer patient.

Richard J. Goldberg, MD

Adv. psychosom. Med., vol. 18, pp. 1–12 (Karger, Basel 1988)

Assessment and Management of the Cancer Patient with Depression

Mary Jane Massie, Jimmie C. Holland

Psychiatry Service, Department of Neurology, Memorial Sloan-Kettering Cancer Center, New York, N.Y.; Department of Psychiatry, Cornell University Medical College, New York, N.Y., USA

The diagnosis of cancer causes stress on any individual which relates both to symptoms of the disease and to the psychologic meaning attached to cancer. The patient's ability to manage these stresses depends on prior level of emotional adjustment, the threat the cancer poses to attainment of age-appropriate goals (e.g. career, starting a family), the presence of emotionally supportive persons in the environment and variables determined by the disease itself (disabling symptoms, site of cancer, treatments required, presence of pain, and prognosis) [17]. When emotional distress associated with having cancer exceeds what is 'expected' or 'normal' a psychiatric disorder may have developed and should be assessed. By far the most common problem seen is depression related to adjusting to cancer. No aspect of the psychological state is more difficult to assess than depression, yet none is more important for the clinician to be able to evaluate. Recognition of pathological levels of depression for which a consultation is needed and for which treatment should be instituted is a critical aspect of patient care. This chapter reviews the prevalence of depression in cancer patients, the types of depressive syndromes, assessment and management principles.

Prevalence of Depression

The prevalence of affective disorder is estimated to be 6% [33]. Thus, a small number of cancer patients can be expected to have the preexisting affective disorder which places them at increased risk of depression during the course of cancer. Two studies by Plum and Holland [30, 31] have indeed confirmed the presence of a history of prior depressive illness among a group of seriously depressed patients with cancer.

The frequency of depression in cancer patients has been the subject of several studies [4, 6, 10, 16, 21, 22] which report rates as high as 58% [16] to as low as 4.5% [22]. Higher frequencies of depression are reported in studies which: (1) depend upon clinician reports of depressive symptoms with the absence of defined diagnostic criteria for depression; (2) include patients with advanced stages of disease, and (3) include patients with more severe levels of illness. The factor with the strongest relationship to clinical depression is physical performance status usually measured by the Karnofsky Scale [20].

Bukberg et al. [4] have conducted the most extensive study to date of depression in hospitalized cancer patients. Using both criteria from the Diagnostic and Statistical Manual-III [7], which were modified to eliminate physical symptoms characteristic of cancer, and validated observer rating scales (Hamilton Rating Scale, Beck Depression Inventory), they found that 24% of the 62 patients studied were severely depressed, 18% moderately depressed, 14% had some depressive symptoms. Forty-four percent showed no depression at all, despite their being hospitalized for treatment in a cancer research hospital. The factor most significantly related to presence of severe depression was the level of physical function: 77% of those most depressed were also the most physically impaired.

Derogatis et al. [6] and Lansky et al. [22] report the lowest rates of affective disorders in cancer patients (13 and 4.5%, respectively). In both of these studies, predefined criteria for the diagnosis of major depression and adjustment disorder with depressed mood were utilized in a patient population which included ambulatory patients with good physical performance status.

In the past depression was generally thought to be greater in patients with cancer than in those with other medical illnesses. Two studies of patients on general medical floors found a similar prevalence of depression, suggesting that cancer patients are no more or less depressed than equally physically ill patients with other diseases [28, 36].

Using criteria from the Diagnostic and Statistical Manual-III classification of psychiatric disorders, the Psychosocial Collaborative Oncology Group in three cancer centers determined psychiatric disorders in 215 randomly accessed hospitalized and ambulatory adult patients with cancer [6]. Slightly over half (53%) of the patients evaluated were adjusting normally to the stress of illness; however, nearly half (47%) had clinically apparent psychiatric disorders. Of these, over two thirds (68%) had adjustment disorder with depressed, anxious or mixed mood; 13% had a major depression; 8%, an organic brain syndrome; 7%, personality disorder, and 4%, anxiety disorder. In general, adjustment disorder with depressed mood and major depression constituted the most frequent diagnoses.

We have reviewed data on 546 patients referred for psychiatric consultation at Memorial Hospital [25]. Of these consultations, 59% had been requested for evaluation of depression or suicidal risk, or both. When the consultants' actual impressions were reviewed, depressive symptoms were by far the most common with adjustment disorders accounting for 54% and major depression 9%.

Clinical Picture

The normal response to hearing the diagnosis of cancer is sadness about loss of health as well as anticipated losses including death. This normal response is part of a spectrum of depressive symptoms which range from normal sadness to adjustment disorder with depressed mood to major depression. There are gradations in 'normal' levels of depressive symptoms. Symptoms vary from minimal when stresses are few, to severe when crises related to illness occur. If symptoms worsen and interfere with daily activity, adjustment disorder with depressed mood is diagnosed. If this reactive state evolves, then criteria for major depression may be met.

With data from studies and extensive clinical observation, it is now possible to predict which patients are at higher risk of depression. The factors which increase the risk of depression are previous history of affective disorder, alcoholism, advanced disease [18], and poorly controlled pain [24].

Cancer patients frequently become depressed at major stress points during cancer: at the time of diagnosis, at time of relapse or general worsening of the patient's condition, and when new treatments must be initiated [17]. Learning that standard cancer treatments are no longer effective is demoralizing and difficult for many patients to accept. Completing a series of treatments (e.g. chemotherapy or radiotherapy) is also stressful for patients who have felt comforted knowing the physician and his staff have been carefully monitoring their progress through a course of treatment [19].

The clinical evaluation includes careful assessment of symptoms, mental status, physical status, treatment effects, and laboratory data. The clinician obtains a history of previous depressive episodes, family history of depression or suicide, concurrent life stress, and availability of social support. An assessment of the meaning of illness to the patient and his understanding of his medical situation is essential. In our experience, the dexamethasone suppression test (DST) and the thyrotropin-releasing hormone (TRH) test are not useful as screening tests for depression in cancer patients.

The diagnosis of depression in physically healthy patients depends heavily on the presence of somatic (vegetative) symptoms of anorexia, fatigue, weight loss, insomnia and anhedonia. These indicators are, however, of little value as diagnostic criteria for depression in cancer patients, since they are common to both cancer and depression. In cancer patients, the diagnosis of depression must depend not on somatic symptoms but on psychologic symptoms, such as dysphoric mood, loss of self-esteem, feelings of helplessness, worthlessness or guilt, difficulty concentrating, and thoughts of 'wishing for death' or suicide.

Early symptoms of delirium (withdrawal or agitation, apathy, and mood lability) and symptoms of mild dementia are often misinterpreted by medical and nursing staff as being symptoms of depression. Psychiatric consultation is often requested to help differentiate these disorders. Likewise, psychiatric consultants are often asked to evaluate the mental state of the cancer patient with pain. Psychiatric symptoms of patients who are in pain must initially be considered as a consequence of uncontrolled pain. Depression with despair (especially when the patient believes the pain means disease progression), agitation, irritability, uncooperativeness, anger, acute anxiety, and inability to sleep are common emotional and behavioral symptoms of pain. These symptoms are not labeled as a psychiatric disorder unless they persist after pain is adequately controlled. Psychiatrists should first assist in pain control and then reassess the patient's mental state after pain is controlled to determine whether the patient has a psychiatric disorder [24].

If a patient has a medical condition or is being treated with medications that are known to cause depression, attempt is first made to treat these disorders. Many metabolic, nutritional, endocrine and neurologic disorders produce symptoms which can be mistaken for depression [14]. Cancer patients with abnormal levels of serum potassium, sodium, or calcium may appear depressed, as can patients who are febrile, anemic or who have vitamin (folate, B_{12}) deficiency. Hypothyroidism, hyperparathyroidism and adrenal insufficiency must be considered in the differential diagnosis of the depressed cancer patient.

Numerous medications can produce symptoms of depression: methyldopa, reserpine, barbiturates, diazepam, and estrogens. Of the many cancer chemotherapeutic agents, depressive symptoms are produced by relatively few: vincristine, vinblastine, procarbazine, *L*-asparaginase, amphotericin B, interferon [38, 40]. The glucocorticosteroids, prednisone and dexamethasone, widely used in cancer as a critical component of standard treatments, in cancer pain management, and to reduce edema from brain and spinal cord tumors, can cause psychiatric disturbances ranging from minor mood disturbances to steroid psychosis. Mood changes resulting from steroids include emotional lability, a sense of well-being, euphoria or depression, sometimes with suicidal ideation [15]. Depressive symptoms resulting from cancer chemotherapy and steroids can be severe, and since continuation of the drugs causing depression is usually absolutely necessary, the psychiatrist often treats these symptoms with antidepressants (see below).

Management

The cornerstone of optimal management for the patient with cancer is the continued emotional support given by the physician with whom the patient has a trusting relationship. Psychiatric consultation should be considered when depressive symptoms last longer than a week, when they worsen rather than improve or when they interfere with the patient's ability to function or to cooperate with treatment. Depressed patients are usually treated with a combination of psychotherapy and antidepressants.

The psychotherapy most often used is a short-term supportive treatment based on a crisis intervention model. In general, the aims of interventions are to increase morale and self-esteem while decreasing distress and improving coping methods or strategies. The goals of psychotherapy are to help the patient regain his sense of self-worth, to correct misconceptions about the past and present and to integrate the present illness into a continuum of life experiences. The patient becomes aware of and must adjust to the fact that plans for the future must often be modified and limitations accepted. Psychotherapy emphasizes past strengths, supports previously successful ways of coping, and mobilizes inner resources. Four to ten sessions are usually sufficient to reduce acute symptoms to a tolerable level, but the length of therapy must be tailored to an individual patient's needs. Including a family member in some of the therapy sessions and having the patient attend a group with others who share similar problems are also beneficial approaches. Prolonged and severe symptoms usually require treatment which combines psychotherapy with somatic treatments (medication or, rarely, electroconvulsive therapy).

The family of the depressed cancer patient (discussed elsewhere in this book, chapter 7) is often distressed by the patient's depressive symptoms, perceiving the patient to have 'given up' or believing symptoms of depression indicate the cancer is worsening. Family members, as well as the patient, need to hear the psychiatrist explain both the biological (if present) and psychological factors contributing to the depressed mood, plans for interventions and the anticipated timing of response to treatment. Since continued family support is essential for the patient's well-being, the psychiatrist will need to inform, encourage and reassure the family.

Most depressed cancer patients are treated as outpatients or on medical oncology units if they are hospitalized for cancer treatment; rarely is transfer to a psychiatric unit necessary or feasible. In most psychiatric hospitals, inpatient facilities are for physically healthy, ambulatory patients and the acutely medically ill cancer patient cannot receive the specialized cancer care he needs.

The cancer patient who has had a depressive episode prior to or during cancer illness should receive special monitoring by the oncologist throughout cancer treatment. If symptoms of depression recur, the patient should be rapidly referred for psychiatric consultation.

Suicide in the Cancer Patient

Suicidal ideation always requires careful assessment to determine whether talk of suicide is a symptom of depression or whether such talk is one way the patient expresses his wish to have ultimate control over intolerable symptoms. Breitbart [2] has recently summarized the vulnerability factors that contribute to high suicide potential. Cancer patients who are at higher risk of suicide are those with poor prognosis or advanced stages of illness, with a prior psychiatric history (including a history of alcohol abuse), a history of previous attempts or a family history of suicide. In addition, the recent death of friends or spouse, few social supports, depression, particularly when hopelessness is a key feature, poorly controlled pain, delirium, and recently having been given information about a grave prognosis are significant risk factors.

In reviewing our findings on consultation requests at Memorial Hospital, only a small percentage of hospitalized cancer patients (3%) seen in consultation were felt to be at high enough risk of suicide attempt to necessitate starting suicide precautions. If suicidal risk is present in a hospitalized cancer patient, we arrange for 24-hour nursing companions to monitor suicide risk and provide continued observation of and support for the patient. Need for companions is reevaluated daily, and one-to-one observation is discontinued when it is no longer necessary.

Suicide attempts in the hospital in the absence of a confusional state are rare. Suicidal acts, if they occur, are more likely to occur in patients with poorly controlled pain, few social supports, and a history of impulsive behavior or underlying emotional problems.

Survivors of the cancer patient who commits suicide should be the subject of careful monitoring and vigorous offer of support. Survivors often have conflicts relating to guilt and anger, even when the suicide of a cancer patient appears to have been 'rational'.

Pharmacologic Management of Depression

There are several reports of the efficacy of antidepressants in depressed patients with serious physical disorders [23, 35]. Our clinical experience supports the usefulness of antidepressants in cancer patients with major depression [26, 27]. The antidepressant agents that can be considered for use in cancer patients are: (1) the tricyclics; (2) 'second-generation' antidepressants; (3) monoamine oxidase inhibitors (MAOI); (4) sympathomimetic stimulants; (5) lithium carbonate, and (6) the triazolobenzodiazepine, alprazolam [24]. Table I shows the starting dose and range of therapeutic daily doses for these drugs.

Tricyclic Antidepressants (Amitriptyline, Imipramine, Doxepin, etc.). The antidepressants most frequently used in the oncology setting are the tricyclic antidepressants (TCA). They are started at a low dose, especially in debilitated patients, beginning with 10–25 mg given at bedtime and increasing the dose by 25 mg every 1–2 days until beneficial effect is achieved. For reasons that are unclear, depressed cancer patients often show a therapeutic response to a tricyclic at much lower doses (25–125 mg q.d.) than are usually required in physically healthy, depressed patients (150–300 mg). Patients are usually maintained on a TCA for 4–6 months after symptoms improve, after which time the dose is gradually lowered and discontinued [32].

The choice of tricyclic depends on the nature of the depressive symptoms, medical problems present, and side effects of the TCA. The depressed patient who is agitated and has insomnia will benefit from the use of a TCA that has sedating effects, such as amitriptyline or doxepin. Patients with

Table I. Antidepressant medications used in cancer patients

Generic name	Starting daily dosage, mg (p.o.)	Therapeutic daily dosage, mg (p.o.)
Tricyclic antidepressants		
Amitriptyline	10–25	75–150
Doxepin	50	75–150
Imipramine	25	75–150
Desipramine	25	75–150
Nortripyline	10–25	100–150
Second-generation antidepressants		
Trazodone	50	150–250
Maprotiline	25	50– 75
Amoxapine	25	100–150
Monoamine oxidase inhibitors		
Isocarboxazid	10	20–40
Phenelzine	15	30–60
Tranylcypromine	10	20–40
Lithium carbonate	300	600–1200
Sympathomimetic stimulants		
Dextroamphetamine	2.5 twice daily	5–10
Methylphenidate	5 twice daily	5–20
Benzodiazepine		
Alprazolam	0.25–1.00	0.75–6.00

psychomotor slowing will benefit from use of the compounds with the least sedating effects, such as protriptyline or desipramine. The patient who has stomatitis secondary to chemotherapy or radiotherapy, or who has slow intestinal motility or urinary retention, should receive a TCA with the least anticholinergic effects, such as desipramine or nortriptyline.

Amitriptyline, imipramine, and doxepin can be given intramuscularly to patients unable to take medications by mouth. Although TCA have not yet been approved for intravenous use in the USA, several studies from Europe indicate their efficacy and safety by this route [5, 29, 37].

Imipramine, doxepin, and amitriptyline are increasingly used in the management of pain in cancer patients with a starting dose of 10–25 mg at bedtime. While the initial assumption was that analgesic effect resulted indirectly from the effect on depression, it is now clear that these tricyclics have a separate specific analgesic action probably mediated through several neurotransmitters, most prominently serotonin.

Second-Generation Antidepressants. If a patient has been given a trial of tricyclic antidepressants without therapeutic effect, or if he cannot tolerate side effects, one of the 'second-generation' antidepressants should be considered: trazodone, amoxapine, or maprotiline. The starting dose and daily therapeutic dosage of these agents vary depending on the compound (table I). Like the tricyclic compounds, the second-generation antidepressants vary in their antihistaminic and anticholinergic effects.

Lithium Carbonate. Patients who have been receiving lithium carbonate for bipolar afffective disorder prior to cancer should be maintained on it throughout cancer treatment, although close monitoring is necessary in the preoperative and postoperative periods when fluids and salt may be restricted. Maintenance dose of lithium may need reduction in seriously ill patients. Lithium should be prescribed with caution for patients receiving cisplatin due to potential nephrotoxicity of both drugs.

There are several reports in the literature regarding the potential usefulness of lithium carbonate for prevention of steroid-induced mood changes [11, 13]. We have not found this use of lithium helpful in preventing steroid psychosis and prefer to use antidepressants and antipsychotics if symptoms appear.

Monoamine Oxidase Inhibitors. If a patient has responded well to an MAOI for depression prior to treatment for cancer, its continued use is warranted. However, most psychiatrists are reluctant to start depressed cancer patients on MAOI because the need for dietary restriction is poorly received by patients who already have dietary and nutritional deficiencies secondary to cancer illness and treatment.

Psychostimulants. The psychostimulants, dextroamphetamine and methylphenidate, are sometimes prescribed for depressed medically ill patients in whom TCA are contraindicated [3, 39]. Dextroamphetamine is also used to potentiate the analgesic effect and counter the sedative effects of narcotics. A common starting dose is 2.5 mg of dextroamphetamine or 5 mg of methylphenidate given at 8 a.m. and noon. Psychostimulants in low dose stimulate appetite and promote a sense of 'well-being'.

Benzodiazepines. The triazolobenzodiazepine alprazolam has been shown to be an effective antidepressant as well as an anxiolytic [12, 34]. Alprazolam is particularly useful in cancer patients who have mixed symptoms of anxiety and depression. Starting dose is 0.25 mg t.i.d.; effective doses are usually in the range of 4–6 mg daily.

Electroconvulsive Therapy

Occasionally electroconvulsive therapy (ECT) is given to depressed cancer patients. The efficacy of ECT has been established most convincingly for the treatment of delusional and severe endogenous depressions. ECT is not effective for patients with milder depression, such as dysthymic disorder or adjustment disorder with depressed mood. Unfortunately ECT still has an unfavorable reputation in the general public and, in our experience, severely physically ill cancer patients (and their families) are often extremely reluctant to consider this form of therapy. Depressed cancer patients in whom ECT should be considered are: (1) those with life-threatening depression (delusional or endogenous depressions) with symptoms which include the refusal to eat, mutism, severe suicidal ideation; (2) those who have responded well to ECT in the past; (3) those who are unable to tolerate the side effects of antidepressant medication or in whom antidepressants are ineffective [1, 8, 9]. Six to twelve treatments are usually effective; the usual frequency of treatment is three times weekly. Following ECT most patients are maintained on tricyclics or lithium to reduce relapse.

References

1 Bidder, T.G.: Electroconvulsive therapy in the medically ill patient. Psychiat. Clin. N. Am. *4:* 391–405 (1981).
2 Breitbart, W.: Suicide in cancer patients. Oncology *1:* 49–53 (1987).
3 Bruera, E.; MacDonald, N.; Chadwick, S.; Brenneis, C.: Double-blind cross-over study of methylphenidate with narcotics for the treatment of cancer pain. Proc. Am. Soc. Clinical Oncology, 987, Abstract, p. 253 (1986).
4 Bukberg, J.; Penman, D.; Holland, J.C.: Depression in hospitalized cancer patients. Psychosom. Med. *46:* 199–212 (1984).
5 Carton, M.; Cabarrot, E.; Lafforque, C.: Intérêt de l'amitriptyline utilisée comme antalgique en cancérologie. (The value of amitriptyline as an analgesic in cancer.) Gaz. med. Fr. *83:* 2375–2378 (1976).
6 Derogatis, L.R.; Morrow, G.R.; Fetting, J.; Penman, D.; Piasetsky, S.; Schmale,

A.M.; Hendricks, M.; Carnicke, C.L.: The prevalence of psychiatric disorders among cancer patients. J. Am. med. Ass. *249:* 751–757 (1983).

7 Diagnostic and Statistical Manual of Mental Disorders; 3rd ed. (Am. Psychiatric Ass., Washington 1981).

8 Dubovsky, S.L.: Using electroconvulsive therapy for patients with neurological disease. Hosp. Comm. Psych. *37:* 819–825 (1986).

9 National Institute of Mental Health: Electroconvulsive therapy. Consensus Development Conf. Statement, vol. 5, No. 11 (1985).

10 Evans, D.L.; McCartney, C.F.; Nemeroff, C.B.; Raft, D.; Quade, D.; Golden, R.N.; Haggerty, J.J.; Holmes, V.; Simon, J.S.; Droba, M.; Mason, G.A.; Fowler, W.C.: Depression in women treated for gynecological cancer: clinical and neuroendocrine assessment. Am. J. Psychiat. *143:* 447–452 (1986).

11 Falk, W.E.; Mahnke, M.W.; Poskanzer, D.C.: Lithium prophylaxis of corticotropin-induced psychosis. J. Am. med. Ass. *241:* 1011–1012 (1979).

12 Feighner, J.P.; Aden, G.C.; Fabre, L.F.; et al.: Comparison of alprazolam, imipramine and placebo in the treatment of depression. J. Am. med. Ass. *249:* 3057–3064 (1983).

13 Goggans, F.C.; Weisberg, L.J.; Koran, L.M.: Lithium prophylaxis of prednisone psychosis: a case report. J. clin. Psychiat. *44:* 111–112 (1983).

14 Hall, R.C.W.; Popkin, M.K.; Devaul, R.A.; Faillace, L.A.; Stickney, S.K.: Physical illness presenting as psychiatric disease. Archs gen. Psychiat. *35:* 1315–1320 (1978).

15 Hall, R.C.W.; Popkin, M.K.; Stickney, S.K.; et al.: Presentation of the steroid psychosis. J. nerv. ment. Dis. *167:* 229–236 (1979).

16 Hinton, J.: Psychiatric consultation in fatal illness. Proc. R. Soc. Med. *65:* 29–32 (1972).

17 Holland, J.C.: Psychological aspects of cancer; in Holland, Frei, Cancer medicine; 2nd ed., pp. 1175–1203, 2325–2331 (Lea & Febiger, Philadelphia 1982).

18 Holland, J.C.; Hughes-Korzun, A.; Tross, S.; Silberfarb, P.; Perry, M.; Cosmis, R.; Oster, M.: Comparative psychological disturbance in pancreatic and gastric cancer. Am. J. Psychiat. *143:* 982–986 (1986).

19 Holland, J.C.; Rowland, J.; Lebovits, A.; Rusalem, R.: Reactions to cancer treatment. Assessment of emotional response to adjuvant radiotherapy as a guide to planned intervention. Psychiat. Clin. N. Am. *2:* 347–358 (1979).

20 Karnofsky, P.A.: Clinical evaluation of anticancer drugs; in Goldin et al., Cancer chemotherapy (Japanese Cancer Ass., Tokyo 1968).

21 Koenig, R.; Levin, S.M.; Brennan, M.J.: The emotional status of cancer patient as measured by a psychological test. J. chron. Dis. *20:* 923–930 (1967).

22 Lansky, S.B.,; List, M.A.; Herrmann, C.A.; Ets-Hokin, E.G.; DasGupta, T.K.; Wilbanks, G.D.; Hendrickson, F.R.: Absence of major depressive disorder in female cancer patients. J. clin. Oncol. *3:* 1553–1560 (1985).

23 Lipsey, J.R.; Robinson, R.G.; Pearlson, G.D., et al.: Nortriptyline treatment of post-stroke depression: a double-blind study. Lancet *i:* 297–300 (1984).

24 Massie, M.J.; Holland, J.C.: The cancer patient with pain: psychiatric complications and their management. Med. Clins N. Am. *71:* 243–258 (1987).

25 Massie, M.J.; Holland, J.C.: Consultation and liaison issues in cancer care. Psychiat. Med. (in press).

26 Massie, M.J.; Holland, J.C.: Current concepts in psychiatric oncology; in Greenspan, Psychiatric update. III, pp. 239–256 (Am. Psychiatric Ass., Washington 1984).

27 Massie, M.J.; Holland, J.C.: Diagnosis and treatment of depression in the cancer patient. J. clin. Psychiat. *45:* 25–28 (1984).
28 Moffic, H.; Paykel, E.S.: Depression in medical inpatients. Br. J. Psychiat. *126:* 346–353 (1975).
29 Mucha, H.; Lange, E.; Bonitz, G.: Amitriptylin in der psychiatrischen Therapie. (Amitriptyline in psychiatric therapy.) Psychiatrie Neurol. med. Psychol. *22:* 116–120 (1970).
30 Plumb, M.; Holland, J.C.: Comparative studies of psychological function in patients with advanced cancer. I. Self-reported depressive symptoms. Psychosom. Med. *39:* 264–276 (1977).
31 Plumb, M.M.; Holland, J.C.: Comparative studies of psychological function in patients with advanced cancer. II. Interviewer-rated current and past psychological symptoms. Psychosom. Med. *43:* 243–254 (1981).
32 Prien, R.F.; Kupfer, D.J.: Continuation drug therapy for major depressive episodes. How long should it continue? Am. J. Psychiat. *143:* 18–23 (1986).
33 Reiger, D.A.; Myers, J.K.; Kramer, M.; Robins, L.N.; Blazer, D.G.; Hough, R.L.; Eaton, W.W.; Locke, B.Z.: The NIMH Epidemiologic Catchment Area Program. Archs gen. Psychiat. *41:* 934–941 (1984).
34 Rickels, K.; Feighner, J.P.; Smith, W.T.: Alprazolam, amitriptyline, doxepine, and placebo in the treatment of depression. Archs gen. Psychiat. *42:* 134–141 (1985).
35 Rifkin, A.; Reardon, G.; Siris, S.; Karagji, B.; Kim, Y.; Hackstaff, L.; Endicott, N.: Trimipramine in physical illness with depression. J. clin. Psychiat. *46:* 4–8 (1985).
36 Schwab, J.J.; Bialow, M.; Brown, J.M.; Holzer, C.E.: Diagnosing depression in medical inpatients. Ann. intern. Med. *67:* 695–707 (1967).
37 Sutter, J.M.; Delpretti, G.M.; Scoitto, J.C.; et al.: Accroissement de l'action antidépressive de l'amitriptyline par la technique des perfusions intra-veineuses. (Increase in the antidepressant effect of amitriptyline by use of intravenous infusion.) Annls. méd.-psychol. *126:* 601–605 (1968).
38 Weddington, W.W.: Delirium and depression associated with amphotericin B. Psychosomatics *23:* 1076–1078 (1982).
39 Woods, S.W.; Tesar, G.E.; Murray, G.B.; Cassem, N.H.: Psychostimulant treatment of depressive disorders secondary to medical illness. J. clin. Psychiat. *47:* 12–15 (1986).
40 Young, D.F.: Neurological complications of cancer chemotherapy; in Silverstein, Neurological complications of therapy: selected topics, pp. 57–113 (Futura, New York 1982).

Mary Jane Massie, MD, Psychiatry Service, 1275 York Avenue,
New York, NY 10021 (USA)

Adv. psychosom. Med., vol. 18, pp. 13–25 (Karger, Basel 1988)

The Effects of Cancer Therapies on the Central Nervous System

Peter M. Silberfarb, Thomas E. Oxman

Department of Psychiatry, Dartmouth Medical School and the Norris Cotton Cancer Center, Dartmouth Hitchcock Medical Center, Hanover, N.H., USA

Introduction

The psychiatric manifestations of cancer therapy on the central nervous system (CNS) can vary from mild focal impairment of intellectual functioning to the global impairment of toxic psychosis or dementia. To adequately detect and treat these effects it is important to have an understanding of cognitive (or intellectual) functioning and the effect that impairment of this functioning has on behavior.

Cognitive functioning, thinking, and intellectual functioning are terms used synonymously in this discussion to indicate the global integrity of one's intellect: the integration of information processing. This integration includes awareness, attention, orientation, memory, perception, comprehension, and abstraction. These are the higher integrative functions of the brain. Defects in these functions can be measured objectively by the standard psychiatric mental status examination or by the many cognitive function tests that have been summarized elsewhere [1].

Impairment of cognitive functioning can be subtle in cancer patients but still is a reflection of abnormalities in cerebral physiology or structure. Cancer patients, as a group, are often older, may have metastases, or suffer from fever, infection, nutritional deficiencies, metabolic or endocrinological abnormalities, or may have a history of risk factors for certain types of cancer, such as alcohol or drug abuse, or be immobilized (bedridden), all of which either predispose or facilitate the individual to the occurrence of impaired cognition. In addition, humans are living longer than they did in the past, whether they have cancer or not, so they are more likely to reach an age where they may be more susceptible to cognitive deficits if challenged by any number of stresses.

Since the problem of cognitive impairment is a spectrum ranging from the subtle to the dramatic, the impairment is often missed by the clinician when 'mild'. The subtle loss of cognitive flexibility, such as being able to sequentially order alternating numbers and letters (as measured by the Trails B Test), the subtle decrease in comprehension of written or spoken instructions, the subtle loss of the ability to think abstractly, the subtle impairment of attention or awareness of one's surroundings, all are often missed by the examining physician. In addition, patients are often able to overcome the deficits, if mild, by heightening their awareness or by devoting more of their energies to these crucial mental functions that, in times of health, are done automatically with minimal intellectual energy. It has been more than 25 years since Engel and Romano [2] demonstrated that impaired cognitive functioning can be objectively measured by the mental status examination and can be correlated with relative slowing of the electroencephalogram and, thus, presumably reflect abnormalities in cerebral physiology. Unfortunately, when these changes are mild, they are often rationalized by both health professional and patient as reflecting anxiety or depression. These symptoms of 'mental fatigue' or difficulty concentrating or increased irritability may, in fact, be the mild prodromata of delirium [3].

It is difficult to judge how frequently cognitive deficits occur in cancer patients generally, much less in those receiving cancer therapies. One reason is that until recently there was no agreement on a classification and, thus, much of the oncology literature does not use the current Psychiatry DSM-III [4] classification when describing neuropsychiatric disorders generally and disorders of cognition specifically. Clinical reports often use words such as confusion, toxic psychosis, mental changes, neurotoxicity, neuropsychiatric side effects, etc. when describing impairments of cognition. This confusion of nosology plus the vexing problem of diagnosing subtle or mild impairment because of the propensity of attributing these deficits to purely behavioral, i.e. psychological etiologies, make judgments about the prevalence of the psychiatric effects of cancer therapies tentative [5].

Despite these difficulties, it is important for all health professionals to be aware of the negative effects that impaired thinking can cause either by the cancer itself or the therapy for cancer. The whole issue of quality of life and the importance of maintaining this for as long as possible need no further elaboration. The simple fact that many of the causes of impaired cognition can be reduced or eliminated is another reason why those caring for cancer patients must be alert to the early and subtle signs of cognitive impairment. Patients also need to be able to give informed consent and have a reasonable understanding of their diagnosis, the therapy, and any research procedures or protocols that may be offered. Finally, comprehending and adhering to treatment plans and recommendations are more apt to be followed in patients who are cognitively intact.

Because of these reasons, it is crucial that the physician identify cognitive impairment as early as possible in the course of a patient's illness or therapy for that illness. The various assessment methods and techniques for cognitive function in cancer patients is reviewed thoroughly elsewhere [1]. There are a number of brief cognitive screening examinations, standardized mental status examinations, and neuropsychological subtests that can be invoked if the physician has access to tertiary care facilities or a neuropsychological laboratory. The formal bedside mental status examination, however, combined with a clinical history and observation, remains a useful and easily accessible way to diagnose and identify the effects of cancer therapies on the CNS [6]. The cornerstone of all methods of cognitive assessment is a simple, but complete, history of the patient's premorbid personality and past life, plus clinical observation of the patient's behavior both verbal and nonverbal. In addition, a careful discussion of the patient's sleep patterns should be done daily. Sleep disruption is often an early indicator of cognitive impairment. This can be simple reversal of the sleep-wakefulness cycle with insomnia and daytime drowsiness. Slight forgetfulness, difficulty finding the correct word when talking, minor misidentifications of persons or surroundings, difficulty concentrating, subtle changes in psychomotor behavior, such as increased purposeless activity or decreased physical activity, reflecting a 'mental dulling', may be other signs of cognitive impairment that are apparent to the careful observer. These changes, when seen in the setting of a healthy, noncancer individual, could reflect changes of behavior secondary to psychogenic issues. However, in the setting of cancer, impaired cognition, and by implication physiological impairment of the brain, must be the first item considered.

Cognitive Testing

In addition to clinical history and observation, the formal cognitive portion of the mental status examination offers the easiest and most accessible diagnostic tool to the clinician. It is an evaluation of objective behavioral responses that describe the patient's current mental functioning and forms an important baseline for later comparisons. For the detection of cognitive impairment, the patient's orientation, memory, awareness, concentration, attention, and abstraction can easily and objectively be assessed. Orientation can easily be tested by asking the patient the date, the day of the week, etc. Likewise, immediate recall, recent memory, and remote memory are easily tested at the bedside. Serial 7 or 3 subtraction, counting backwards, or digit span retention are used as tests of attention and concentration (not arithmetic ability) that can be obtained in the office or at the bedside. A patient's ability to abstract can be measured by simple proverbs or asking the patient how pairs of objects are similar (similarities). Finally, it is often useful to assess the patient's constructional ability by asking the patient to draw a three-dimensional cube, a two-dimensional cross, or a horizontal diamond.

There are three general principles that the physician must apply when conducting the mental status examination. In order to decrease anxiety and focus concentration within the patient's abilities, the patient should be made to feel as comfortable as possible by stating that this is a routine part of the examination so that the physician can periodically assess the effects of their tumor or treatment on their concentration and memory. Second, encouragement and support by the examiner is appropriate; therefore, the easy questions should be asked before the harder ones. Finally, since a patient is going to be asked these questions periodically to assess his or her functioning (such as digit span), correct answers should not be given except for questions involving orientation.

For patients who are psychologically healthy before the onset of cancer, it is unusual for severe functional psychiatric sequelae to follow the diagnosis of cancer or the treatment of cancer. If symptoms such as these develop, the physician should always consider first one of the organic mental disorders reflected in impaired cognition or a medication-responsive depressive illness. This has been shown for cancer patients generally [7, 8] and specifically breast cancer patients [9, 10] and patients with multiple myeloma [11] to name a few. This observation, however, should not be construed to lessen the importance nor lessen the potential psychological impact of cancer therapies. Common sense and simple observation reveal that emotional suffering is experienced by almost all patients with serious illness, of which cancer is this century's archetype. Even long after cancer therapy has ceased, psychological and social sequelae can persist. Meyerowitz et al. [12] demonstrated this in their follow-up of breast cancer patients almost two years after active cancer therapy had ended. These were disease-free patients who, at follow-up, while reporting significant improvements in quality of life, did report continuing long-term disruption in general activity. The majority of these patients also described continuing physical problems that they related to chemotherapy.

Metastatic Disease

In assessing the occurrence of CNS effects of cancer therapies, the clinician should obviously be aware of the common cancers that are associated most frequently with CNS metastasis. These cancers are: lung, breast, malignant melanoma, and testicular cancers [13]. One study [14] found that impaired cognitive functioning occurred in 77% of 167 cases as the presenting symptom of brain metastasis. Zimm et al. [15] reported impaired cognitive functioning as the presenting symptom of brain metastasis in 35% of their 192 cases of intracerebral metastasis in patients with solid tumors. Only headache, which occurred in 38% of their patients, was more frequent as a presenting symptom than cognitive impairment. Similarly, leptomeningeal carcinoma can present with changes in the mental status examination as its first symptom.

Chemotherapeutic Agents

Many chemotherapeutic agents have been implicated as cancer therapies that cause psychiatric CNS effects [5, 16]. Most chemotherapy, however, is given in protocols combined with other chemotherapeutic agents or with radiation therapy. It is difficult, therefore, to identify a single agent.

Methotrexate is often implicated, alone or in combination with radiotherapy, as a cause of organic brain syndrome. This usually has been associated with prolonged therapy by the intrathecal route and associated with chronic progressive leukoencephalopathy. Recently, however, an encephalopathy that begins abruptly and consists of behavioral abnormalities, ranging from inappropriate laughter to lethargy, has been reported in patients treated for osteogenic sarcoma with high-dose methotrexate followed by leucovorin rescue [17]. Many other chemotherapeutic agents can cause an organic brain syndrome. The vinca alkaloids have been reported to cause 'mental changes', 'hallucinations', 'confusion', and 'delirium' [18–20]. High doses of cytosine arabinoside (ara-C) has been reported to cause confusion and drowsiness in addition to symptoms of cerebellar dysfunction [21, 22]. Donehauer et al. [23] reported dose-related CNS toxicity consisting of somnolence during ara-C infusion. A recent report on the CNS toxicity with high-dose ara-C reported 12% (or 14) of 118 adults being treated for acute leukemia had evidence of encephalopathy and 10 of these experienced confusion, disorientation, memory loss and general cognitive dysfunction [24].

Fludarabine phosphate (FAMP) was used to treat 70 patients with acute leukemia. Eleven of these patients experienced encephalopathy with deterioration of their mental status. In a number of these patients, an electroencephalogram was performed and revealed diffuse slowing correlating with the impaired cognitive function reflected in deteriorating mental status examination [25]. Merkel et al. [26] also reported encephalopathy with fludarabine treatment in a patient with mycosis fungoides.

BCNU (Carmustine), a nitrosourea can produce, either in high doses or in standard doses when combined with radiation, an acute encephalopathy [16]. CCNU has also been cited as a cause of global cognitive impairment when given in combination with brain irradiation [27]. Isophosphamide has been reported to cause disorientation, visual hallucinations, and somnolence by Kovach et al. [28] in 1974. Heime et al. [29] reported psychopathological symptoms in 7 of 10 patients treated for renal carcinoma with this agent. Procarbazine [30], nitrogen mustard [18], and BCNU when given intra-arterially [31] have caused confusion, psychosis, disorientation, or altered levels of consciousness. Greenwald [32], writing in the Journal of the American Medical Association in 1976, reported mental changes typical of delirium with disorientation and slowing of the electroencephalogram in patients being treated with fluorouracil. Ftorafur, an analog of 5-fluorouracil, has been reported as causing confusion and forgetfulness when used in combination with CCNU [33]. *L*-Asparaginase is a well-known cause of cognitive impairment [34].

Several chemotherapeutic agents that may cause cognitive impairment, as inferred from clinical case reports, are aminoglutethimide [35], DTIC [36] and 5-azacytidine [37]. Steroids, whether used as adjuncts to treatment or as chemotherapeutic agents directly as in the leukemias, lymphomas, or breast cancer with bony metastasis, are well known to cause behavioral symptoms such as euphoria, depression, or psychosis. In cancer patients, steroids are often used to treat hypercalcemia and cerebral edema, both of which can in and of themselves cause mental impairment. Cisplatinum, a frequently used and very toxic chemotherapeutic agent, has been reported to cause encephalopathy when used by means of the intracarotid infusion [38]. Hexamethylmelamine has been reported to cause mental depression and hallucinations [34].

Finally, when discussing CNS effects of chemotherapeutic agents, one must also look beyond the direct toxic effects of these agents on cognitive functioning. Respiratory insufficiency such as might be caused by bleomycin, congestive heart failure such as might occur following use of adriamycin, or azotemia following renal damage secondary to cisplatinum are all conditions that are well known to result in encephalopathy.

Interferon

The clinical toxicity of human interferons has recently been reviewed [40]. These agents have antitumor activity in a variety of cancers. Fatigue, which has been called the most important dose-limiting toxic effect of interferon, is often manifested as social withdrawal or job absenteeism. In higher doses both natural or DNA-derived interferons can cause confusion and diffuse slowing of the electroencephalogram consistent with encephalopathy [41]. Psychoses with hallucinations are rare but have been reported [42]. Even in low doses, interferon can produce behavioral changes when patients are assessed with specific neuropsychiatric tests [43, 44]. Abnormal electroencephalograms, agitation, and disorientation have also been reported in patients who have received interferon after bone marrow transplantation. However, these patients were also receiving acyclovir, an antiviral agent, because of herpes virus infections, and it may have been this medication that caused the abnormal findings [45].

Radiation Therapy

Radiation therapy, both alone and in combination with chemotherapy, has been reported to produce neurotoxicity. McMahon and Vahora [46] reviewed radiation damage to the brain from a neuropsychiatric perspective. They present two cases in which cognitive changes and mood disorders were a prominent part of the clinical picture of radiation necrosis of the brain. The adverse effects of brain irradiation have been extensively reviewed in a book edited by Gilbert and Kagan [47] entitled *Radiation Damage to the Nervous System*. Commonly, the adverse effects of irradiation on the brain are typically divided into three groups depending on the time of appearance of the symptoms: acute reactions which occur during the course of irradiation, early delayed reactions which appear from a few weeks to a few months after irradiation, and late delayed reactions. The acute reactions are secondary to cerebral edema and may be accompanied by mild cognitive impairment. The early delayed reactions are thought to be a result of demyelination and generally resolve spontaneously within a few weeks. It is the late delayed reactions, albeit rare, that can cause pathological changes in brain tissues such as leukoencephalopathy with its resultant serious impairment of intellect. Leukoencephalopathies with intellectual deterioration have been reported in adults with lung cancer who have received high-dose brain irradiation without chemotherapy [48], as well as in children receiving cranial radiation for brain tumors [49].

A combination of radiotherapy and chemotherapy has received the most attention as the cause of cognitive impairment in children following treatment of childhood leukemias [50]. Ch'ein et al. [51] reported learning disabilities as a late effect in children with acute lymphocytic leukemia who had received methotrexate and brain radiation. Recently, however, Williams and Davis [52] have reviewed the literature concerning prophylactic radiation treatment from the vantage point of neuropsychological outcome. These authors challenge the view that cranial radiation results in greater cognitive impairment than treatment without radiation, although this study supports the finding that children under the age of 8 have a worse outcome than children who are older. In adults, prophylactic brain radiation has been employed in the treatment of small cell lung cancer patients who were receiving procarbazine and methotrexate. These patients were at a higher risk for central neurotoxicity than those without brain radiation [48]. Another study [53] reported diffuse encephalopathy in 7 of 49 patients with small cell carcinoma of the lung who had received various combinations of chemotherapeutic agents plus prophylactic brain irradiation.

Other Untoward Effects of Treatment

Side effects and complications of therapy such as pain, nausea and vomiting, infections of the CNS, and secondary CNS tumors are all possible effects of cancer therapies on the CNS. Generally, pain as a consequence of cancer therapy is usually of short duration and easily managed. However, occasionally severe and chronic pain syndromes can occur as a complication of cancer treatments. It is difficult to assess how frequently pain of this type occurs or is related to specific therapies. The muscle and bone pain observed in patients receiving ara-C is one such example, as is the peripheral neuropathy that occurs, on occasion, after therapy with vincristine. Nor is the problem limited to chemotherapy. Radiation-induced enteritis or the pain syndromes that can follow radical neck dissection or mastectomy are examples of treatment-related complications. Pain in cancer patients as a consequence of therapy has been reviewed by Schreml [54]. Pain, of course, is a common problem for patients with cancer, especially those with metastatic disease. And pain relief in patients with cancer continues to be a problem because of undermedication [55]. Virtually all the medications used to treat pain can cause cognitive impairment. Behavioral medicine techniques may be less toxic in this regard. Nausea and vomiting are common side effects of many forms of cancer therapy especially, but not limited to, chemotherapeutic agents. Cisplatin and cyclophosphamide are only two such offenders. Steroids such as dexamethasone or methylprednisolone and metoclopramide have been used as antiemetic agents and have been reported to cause CNS effects such as 'nervousness' [56]. Antiemetics such as the cannabinoids cause CNS effects such as confusion or mood disorders [57] especially when used in doses necessary to produce the antiemetic effect.

Finally, the CNS infections that often follow cancer treatment in the immunocompromised patient can result in meningoencephalitis or brain abscesses. In this situation the organisms are often rather predictable, whether they be bacteria, fungi, parasites or viruses. A delirium or other behavioral disorder reflecting cognitive impairment, often initially subtle, are frequent first manifestations of these infections.

Conclusion and Future Directions

Over the past decade we have seen an increase in the use of cancer therapies and the techniques of delivering these therapies that involve both increasingly toxic agents, massive doses of these toxic agents, and an increasing use of coordinated multimodality therapies, for example, the combined use of surgery, irradiation, and chemotherapy. Many of these protocols have resulted in a marked improvement of survival. Nowhere is this more dramatic than in the multimodality therapies used in the treatment of children with cancer. These treatments, however, have both short-term and long-term complications. The early complications of therapies are fairly well known and, over the past half a decade, the delayed consequences of these rigorous therapies have become apparent. D'Angio [58] divides the late effects of treatment into two broad categories: oncogenesis and functional impairment. The latter most often affects the reproductive system and the CNS. The well-documented delayed consequences of combined brain irradiation plus intrathecal and systemic methotrexate is the most well-known example of the latter which results in learning and school problems in survivors of childhood leukemia [50]. There are only a few studies, however, in adults that specifically focus on neuropsychiatric impairment [8, 27, 59]. Recently, Marie et al. [60] did specific neuropsychiatric testing on patients post therapy for brain tumor; all had Karnofsky scores equal to or greater than 80% and were disease-free as judged by CT scans at the time of psychometric testing. Patients showed significant intellectual deterioration at 4–5 months post treatment. Specifically, tasks requiring attention and immediate problem-solving ability were done poorly. There was also some evidence that with time some deficits improved.

More recently, the development of the concept of targeted delivery of therapy promises to reduce the toxicity of cancer therapies while maintaining the higher cure rate achieved by toxic and multimodality treatments. Monoclonal antibodies, either because of their direct antitumor effects, or their use as homing devices to specifically guide therapeutic agents to the targeted tissue, offer new hope for less toxic therapeutic intervention. Carrier techniques, such as liposomes or controlled release polymers, offer the possibility of directing therapies to the affected tissues alone, thus avoiding massive toxicity. Mechanical reservoirs and implantable pumps have been used to perfuse the CNS with cancer therapies [61]. Paradoxically, targeted delivery systems, carrier techniques, and mechanical devices, while offering the hope of decreased general toxicity, will be used to disrupt the blood-brain barrier thus attacking the sanctuaries harboring cancer cells which most often are located in the CNS. In effect then, we may, in the future, be seeing an increase in psychiatric side effects of chemotherapies because of the new and more effective techniques utilized by targeted drug delivery systems into the CNS. The physician, more than ever before, must be alert to the increasing occurrence of cognitive impairment in cancer patients.

References

1 Oxman, T.E.; Schnurr, P.P.; Silberfarb, P.M.: Assessment of cognitive function in cancer patients. Hospice J. *2:* 99–128 (1986).

2 Engel, G.L.; Romano, J.: Delirium, a syndrome of cerebral insufficiency. J. chron. Dis. *9:* 260–277 (1959).
3 Lipowski, Z.J.: Delirium: acute brain failure in man. (Thomas, Springfield 1980).
4 Diagnostic and Statistical Manual of Mental Disorders; 3rd ed. (DSM-III) (Am. Psychiatric Ass., Washington 1980).
5 Silberfarb, P.M.: Chemotherapy and cognitive defects in cancer patients. A. Rev. Med. *34:* 35–46 (1983).
6 Roca, R.P.: Bedside cognitive examination. Psychosomatics *28:* 71–76 (1987).
7 Levine, P.M.; Silberfarb, P.M.; Lipowski, Z.J.: Mental disorders in cancer patients: a study of 100 psychiatric referrals. Cancer *43:* 1385–1391 (1978).
8 Silberfarb, P.M.; Philibert, D.; Levine, P.M.: Psychosocial aspects of neoplastic disease. II. Affective and cognitive effects of chemotherapy in cancer patients. Am. J. Psychiat. *137:* 1263–1265 (1980).
9 Silberfarb, P.M.; Maurer, L.H.; Crouthamel, C.S.: Psychosocial aspects of neoplastic disease. I. Functional status of breast cancer patients during different treatment regimens. Am. J. Psychiat. *137:* 450–455 (1980).
10 Bloom, J.R.; Cook, M.; Fotopoulis, S.; Flamer, D.; Gates, C.; Holland, J.C.; Muenz, L.R.; Murawski, B.; Penman, D.; Ross, R.D.: Psychological response to mastectomy. Cancer *59:* 189–196 (1987).
11 Silberfarb, P.M.; Bates, G.M., Jr.: Psychiatric complications of multiple myeloma. Am. J. Psychiat. *140:* 788–789 (1983).
12 Meyerowitz, B.E.; Watkins, I.K.; Sparks, F.C.: Psychosocial implications of adjuvant chemotherapy. Cancer *52:* 1541–1545 (1983).
13 Akman, S.A.; Block, J.B.: Neurologic complications of systemic cancer. Primary Care *11:* 597–623 (1984).
14 Posner, J.B.: Neurologic complications of systemic cancer. Med. Clins N. Am. *63:* 783–800 (1979).
15 Zimm, S.; Wampler, G.L.; Stablein, D.; et al.: Intracerebral metastases in solid tumor patients. Cancer *48:* 384–394 (1981).
16 Shapiro, W.R.; Young, D.F.: Neurological complications of antineoplastic therapy. Acta neurol. scand. *70:* suppl. 100, pp. 125–132 (1984).
17 Walker, R.W.; Allen, J.C.; Rosen, G.; Caparros, B.: Transient cerebral dysfunction secondary to high-dose methotrexate. J. clin. Oncol. *4:* 1845–1850 (1986).
18 Hildebrand, J.: Lesions of the nervous system in cancer patients (Raven, New York 1978).
19 Rosenthal, S.; Kaufman, S.: Vincristine neurotoxicity. Ann. intern. Med. *80:* 733–737 (1974).
20 Ohnuma, T.; Greenspan, E.M.; Holland, J.F.: Initial clinical study with vindesine: tolerance to weekly I.V. bolus and 24-hour infusion. Cancer Treat. Rep. *64:* 25–30 (1980).
21 Nand, S.; Messmore, H.L., Jr.; Patel, R.; Fisher, S.G.; Fisher, R.I.: Neurotoxicity associated with systemic high-dose cytosine arabinoside. J. clin. Oncol. *4:* 571–575 (1986).
22 Lazarus, H.M.; Herzig, R.H.; Herzig, G.P.; Phillips, G.L.; Roessmann, U.; Fishman, D.J.: Central nervous system toxicity of high-dose systemic cytosine arabinoside. Cancer *48:* 2577–2582 (1981).
23 Donehauer, R.C.; Karp, J.E.; Burke, P.J.: Pharmacology and toxicity of high-dose cytarabine by 72-hour continuous infusion. Cancer Treat. Rep. *70:* 1059–1065 (1986).

24 Hwang, T.-L.; Yung, W.K.A.; Estey, E.H.; Fields, W.S.: Central nervous system toxicity with high-dose Ara-C. Neurology *35:* 1475–1478 (1985).
25 Chun, H.G.; Leyland-Jones, B.R.; Caryk, S.M.; Hoyj, D.F.: Central nervous system toxicity of fludarabine phosphate. Cancer Treat. Rep. *70:* 1225–1228 (1986).
26 Merkel, D.E.; Griffin, N.L.; Kagan-Hallet, K.; Von Hoff, D.D.: Central nervous system toxicity with fludarabine. Cancer Treat. Rep. *70:* 1449–1450 (1986).
27 Hochberg, F.H.; Slotnick, B.: Neuropsychiatric impairment in astrocytoma survivors. Neurology *30:* 172–177 (1980).
28 Kovach, J.S.; Schutt, A.J.; Hahn, R.G.; Reitemeier, R.J.; Moertel, C.G.: A phase-2 study of intermittent high-dose isophosphamide therapy of advanced colorectal cancer. Oncology *29:* 34–39 (1974).
29 Heim, M.E.; Feine, R.; Schick, E.; Wolpert, E.; Queisser, W.: Central nervous side effects following ifosfamide monotherapy of advanced renal carcinoma. J. Cancer Res. clin. Oncol. *100:* 113–116 (1981).
30 Weiss, H.D.; Walker, M.D.; Wiernik, P.H.: Neurotoxicity of commonly used antineoplastic agents. New Engl. J. Med. *291:* 75–81 (1974).
31 Madajewicz, S.; West, C.R.; Park, H.C.; Ghoorah, J.; Avellanosa, A.M.; Takita, H.; Karakousis, C.; Vincent, R.; Caracandas, J.; Jennings, E.: Phase II study — intraarterial BCNU therapy for metastatic brain tumor. Cancer *47:* 653–657 (1981).
32 Greenwald, E.S.: Organic mental changes with fluorouracil. J. Am. med. Ass. *235:* 248–249 (1976).
33 Belt, R.J.; Stephens, R.: Phase-II study of ftorafur and methyl-CCNU in advanced colorectal cancer. Cancer *44:* 869–872 (1979).
34 Holland, J.; Fasanello, S.; Ohnuma, T.: Psychiatric symptoms associated with *L*-asparaginase administration. J. psychiat. Res. *10:* 105–113 (1974).
35 Hoffken, K.; Kempf, H.; Miller, A.A.; Miller, B.; Schmidt, C.G.; Faber, P.; Kley, H.K.: Aminoglutethimide without hydrocortisone in the treatment of postmenopausal patients with advanced breast cancer. Cancer Treat. Rep. *70:* 1153–1157 (1986).
36 Paterson, A.H.G.; McPherson, T.A.: A possible neurologic complication of DTIC. Cancer Treat. Rep. *61:* 105–106 (1977).
37 Levy, J.A.; Wiernik, P.H.: A comparative clinical trial of 5-azacytidine and guanazole in previously treated adults with acute nonlymphocytic leukemia. Cancer *38:* 36–41 (1976).
38 Stewart, D.J.; Wallace, S.; Feun, L.; et al.: A phase I study of intracarotid artery infusion of cisdiamminedichloroplatinum(II) in patients with recurrent malignant intracerebral tumors. Cancer Res. *42:* 2059–2062 (1982).
39 Legha, S.S.; Slavik, M.; Carter, S.K.: Hexamethylmelamine — an evaluation of its role in the therapy of cancer. Cancer *38:* 27–35 (1976).
40 Quesada, J.R.; Talpaz, M.; Rios, A.; Kurzrock, R.; Gutterman, J.U.: Clinical toxicity of interferons in cancer patients: a review. J. clin. Oncol. *4:* 234–243 (1986).
41 Mattson, K.; Niranen, A.; Iivanainen, M.; et al.: Neurotoxicity of interferon. Cancer Treat. Rep. *67:* 958–961 (1983).
42 Kirkwood, J.M.; Ernstoff, M.S.; Davis, C.A.; et al.: Comparison of intramuscular and intravenous recombinant alpha-2 interferon in melanoma and other cancers. Ann. intern. Med. *103:* 32–36 (1985).
43 Adams, F.; Quesada, J.R.; Gutterman, J.U.: Neuropsychiatric manifestations of human leukocyte interferon therapy in patients with cancer. J.Am. med. Ass. *252:* 938–941 (1984).

44 Mattson, K.; Niiranen, A.; Laaksonen, et al.: Psychometric monitoring of interferon neurotoxicity. Lancet *i:* 275–276 (1984).

45 Wade, J.C.; Meyers, J.D.: Neurologic symptoms associated with parenteral acyclovir treatment after marrow transplantation. Ann. intern. Med. *98:* 921–925 (1983).

46 McMahon, T.; Vahora, S.: Radiation damage to the brain: neuropsychiatric aspects. Gen. Hosp. Psychiat. *8:* 437–441 (1986).

47 Gilbert, H.A.; Kagan, A.R.(eds): Radiation damage to the nervous system (Raven Press, New York 1980).

48 Lee, Y.-Y.; Nauert, C.; Glass, J.P.: Treatment-related white matter changes in cancer patients. Cancer *57:* 1473–1482 (1986).

49 Duffner, P.K.; Cohen, M.E.; Thomas, P.R.M.; Lansky, S.B.: The long-term effects of cranial irradiation on the central nervous system. Cancer *56:* 1841–1846 (1985).

50 Meadows, A.T.; Evans, A.E.: Effects of chemotherapy on the central nervous system. Cancer *37:* 1079–1085 (1976).

51 Ch'ien, L.T.; Aur, R.J.A.; Stagner, S.; Cavallo, K.; Wood, A.; Goff, J.; Pitner, S.; Hustu, H.O.; Seifert, M.J.; Simone, J.V.: Long-term neurological implications of somnolence syndrome in children with acute lymphocytic leukemia. Ann. Neurol. *8:* 273–277 (1980).

52 Williams, J.M.; Davis, K.S.: Central nervous system prophylactic treatment for childhood leukemia: neuropsychological outcome studies. Cancer Treat. Rev. *13:* 113–127 (1986).

53 Chak, L.Y.; Zatz, L.M.; Wasserstein, P.; Cox, R.S.; Kushlan, P.D.; Porzig, K.J.; Sikic, B.I.: Neurologic dysfunction in patients treated for small cell carcinoma of the lung: a clinical and radiological study. Int. J. Radiat. Oncol. Biol. Phys. *12:* 385–389 (1986).

54 Schreml, W.: Pain in the cancer patient as a consequence of therapy (surgery, radiotherapy, chemotherapy). Cancer Res. *89:* 85–99 (1984).

55 Cleeland, C.S.: The impact of pain on the patient with cancer. Cancer *54:* 2635–2641 (1984).

56 Roila, F.; Tonato, M.; Basurto, C.; Bella, M.; Passalacqua, R.; Morsia, D.; DiCostanzo, F.; Donati, D.; Ballatori, E.; Tognoni, G.; Franzosi, M.G.; Del Favero, A.: Antiemetic activity of high doses of metoclopramide combined with methylprednisolone versus metoclopramide alone in cisplatin-treated cancer patients: a randomized double-blind trial of the Italian oncology group for clinical research. J. clin. Oncol. *5:* 141–149 (1987).

57 Eyre, H.J.; Ward, J.H.: Control of cancer chemotherapy-induced nausea and vomiting. Cancer *54:* 2642–2648 (1984).

58 D'Angio, G.J.: Early and delayed complications of therapy. Cancer *51:* 2515–2518 (1983).

59 Maire, J.P.; Coudin, B.; Demeaux, H.; Celerier, D.; Guerin, J.; Caudry, M.: Incidence probable de l'irradiation cérébrale sur l'efficience intellectuelle. Bull. Cancer *70:* 275–283 (1983).

60 Maire, J.P.; Coudin, B.; Guerin, J.; Caudry, M.: Neuropsychologic impairment in adults with brain tumors. Am. J. clin. Oncol. *10:* 156–162 (1987).

61 Freeman, A.I.; Mayhew, E.: Targeted drug delivery. Cancer *58:* 573–583 (1986).

Peter M. Silberfarb, MD, Department of Psychiatry, Dartmouth Medical School and the Norris Cotton Cancer Center, Dartmouth Hitchcock Medical Center, Hanover, NH 03756 (USA)

Adv. psychosom. Med., vol. 18, pp. 26–36 (Karger, Basel 1988)

Neuropsychiatric Evaluation and Treatment of Delirium in Cancer Patients

Frank Adams

Division of Neuropsychiatric Oncology, Neurobehavioral Center and Pain Service, The Ontario Cancer Institute/The Princess Margaret Hospital, Toronto, Ont., Canada

Introduction

Delirium is a condition of acute cerebral insufficiency resulting from widespread disruption of brain metabolism. The incidence and pathophysiology of delirium remain elusive, but its occurrence in patients with serious illness, such as cancer, is notably high. Because delirium is a frequent prelude to persistent dementia or death, prompt recognition and diagnosis, followed by rapid, effective symptomatic treatment is essential for patient safety, survival and subsequent Quality of Life [1].

Despite its ubiquity, the clinical importance of delirium has been overshadowed by disputes about its clinical existence, its meaning, outcome, and the need to treat. Even where agreement exists on the necessity for treatment, further controversy surrounds method, choice of medications, and routes of administration. Most often, treatment is provided only if the patient's behavior becomes disruptive, at which time medication is given simply for the purpose of restraint [2]. Rational pharmacology at these times is seldom in evidence.

The search for a medically reversible cause is rare. Too often physicians still favor the unsound and far-fetched conclusion that psychologic or psychosocial factors, especially 'understandable' stress play a causal role. The psychosocial model as a general explanation for all changes in patients' moods or behaviors is endemic in oncology [3, 4].

Generally speaking, however, delirium is usually unrecognized or ignored. If addressed at all, it is just as likely to be misdiagnosed as 'depression', 'psychosis', 'hysteria' or 'personality disorder'. This widespread use of vague and nonspecific psychiatric jargon, a major impediment to understanding, evaluating, and effectively treating delirium, all too often substitutes for sound medical reasoning by psychiatrists and oncologists alike.

The agitated delirious cancer patient poses a formidable diagnostic and therapeutic challenge for even the most experienced physician. The disease, its highly toxic treatments, and the concurrent medical complications confound the search for etiology, which more often than not, defies identification. Therefore, a logical and thorough diagnostic approach to the confused brain-impaired cancer patient is essential, and must be combined with an understanding of the pharmacology of the drugs selected for treatment. Psychiatrists who provide consultation services to oncology units also need to be intimately familiar with the neurotoxic effects of the more potent chemotherapeutic agents [5], and the neurologic features of cancer and the brain [6]. For physicians confronted by the protean and complex neuropsychiatric manifestations of brain failure in oncology, this chapter presents an overview of the clinical features of delirium, and the essentials of a method of emergency neuropharmacologic treatment.

Pathogenesis

Establishing pathogenesis with scientific rigor has been an elusive if not impossible task. The major stumbling block has been the lack of understanding of the mechanisms of disruption of brain function, and the relative paucity of scientifically adequate human data. Research on delirium has been hampered by the difficulties inherent in trying to study severely ill patients, and devising appropriate laboratory tests to measure the internal milieu of the living brain. Nonetheless, there is consensus that delirium is a manifestation of generalized cerebral insufficiency, with widespread dysregulation of neurotransmitter systems [2, 7, 8].

Currently favored pathophysiologic mechanisms include: (1) a cholinergic-dopaminergic imbalance; (2) dopamine and β-endorphin hyperfunction; (3) increased central noradrenergic activity, and (4) intraneuronal damage of enzyme systems [9–11]. Selective loss of neuronal populations (especially in the frontal cortex, the hippocampus, and the locus ceruleus) and a decrease in the function of acetylcholine, is thought to account for the increased susceptibility to delirium in the elderly [10]. This is significant because better than 50% of cancer patients are aged 65 and older.

The idea of a unitary mechanism underlying delirium, though tempting, is probably not correct. This may explain in large measure why no single drug has been totally effective in all episodes of delirium, and may account in part for the ongoing controversy about which drug is the best. Unless there is a critical, specific neurotransmitter subserving a final common pathway in those brain centers responsible for delirium, then a single agent regimen seems unlikely to be useful. This would support the multidrug approach currently favored by us [12] and others [13, 14].

Clinical Features

Delirium is a metabolic lesion of the brain, the consequent neurochemical commotion resulting in the bizarre behaviors and symptoms which are so characteristic of the disorder. It is primarily an altered state of consciousness which results in secondary behavioral and cognitive impairments [15]. In the critically ill cancer patient, especially the aged and those with multisystem organ failure, delirium is frequently inevitably progressive [16]. In other cases it is time-limited, but recovery is only partial, and the patient is left demented. In the minority of cases, recovery is complete: It can be spontaneous, the result of appropriate neuroleptic therapy, or follow upon successful treatment of underlying medical causes. Delirium in patients with advanced cancer often heralds the terminal phase of the illness and progresses to coma and death [1, 17]. In fact, delirium is probably the hallmark of dying. Focal or generalized seizures, though possible, are not common.

Delirious patients display some or all of the following: fluctuating periods of restlessness, agitation, and lethargy; varying degrees of orientation, attention, and cognitive functioning; and a mixture of insomnia and hypersomnia, with characteristic reversal of night and day.

Generally, the condition is worse at night, with acceleration of disruptive behavior, frightening and vivid visual hallucinations (frequently of absent or dead relatives and friends), extreme suspiciousness, hostility and even combativeness. Incoherent mumbling, interspersed with loud shouts, multifocal myoclonus, picking at the bedclothes, and aimless arm and leg movements are common. Deliberate and accidental disconnections from intravenous lines and catheters with self-extubation of breathing apparatus further jeopardize the dangerously ill patient. Less florid presentations are usually not noticed by the medical staff who often sympathetically suggest that the quiet, withdrawn patient seems to be 'depressed'.

For the patient the experience is an endless nightmare in which one becomes an unwilling spectator to and victim of ceaseless chaotic neurosensory experiences. Faulty information processing and grotesque perceptual productions are the hallmarks of a brain in a state of chemical anarchy. Voluntary control over the ability to select and shift the focus of one's mental activity is universally impaired, and in severe cases completely lost. The delicate line between reality and surrealistic fantasy is erased by the aberrant neurochemical tides. Thus, catheters become snakes, walls a menacing kaleidoscope of hideous visual apparitions, and nurses torturers and poisoners. Many patients experience short-term auditory memory, concentration, and sleep impairments, and nocturnal flashbacks weeks and months after apparent recovery from the acute event. Irreversible brain damage with persistent dementia in survivors of severe and prolonged delirium is not uncommon and constitutes a tragic legacy for many patients otherwise cured of cancer.

Etiology

The search for etiology is undoubtedly the greatest source of frustration. Contrary to pronouncements in the leading textbooks of psychiatry and neurology, identifying the cause of a patient's delirium and correcting the condition is rarely a common and straightforward matter.

Delirium has long suffered, not from a lack of etiology, but from a surfeit of possible causes. A host of medical and drug complications, to which there seems to be no end, can cause or result in delirium. Most, however, only prove to be accessories to the condition which is largely multifactorial.

Generally speaking, delirium does not have *a* cause. Not only are there a tremendous number of causes, but they are very likely additive in their actions. It seems to be a fundamental rule of delirium that delirogenic agents and events are cumulative. It is therefore difficult, if not impossible, to assign preeminent importance to any single factor in the vast majority of cases, though in cancer patients there are notable critical exceptions to be kept in mind.

These exceptions constitute a significant and important group of not uncommon neurologic disorders whose principal and often only symptom is delirium, and which are frequently treatable. The notable disorders represented in this group are: leptomeningeal disease; treatment-induced leukoencephalopathy; CNS leukemia; both multiple and solitary brain metastases;

hypomagnesemia secondary to intractable nausea and vomiting, especially after cisplatinum therapy; delayed hypothyroidism following irradiation and/or surgery for head and neck cancer; hypercalcemia from extensive bone metastasis; narcotic analgesics, particularly meperidine and methadone; and the neurotoxicities of chemotherapy. Cytosine arabinoside (ara-C), vincristine, interferon, interleukin, ifosfamide, and caracemide are the commonest offenders in this latter group. Recent clinical experience also suggests that all of these compounds can uncover and probably exacerbate unsuspected preexisting neuropathology.

Investigation into cause begins with determination of arterial blood gases, hemograms, thyroid and adrenal function studies, and an exhaustive review of past and current medical treatments and medications. Nurses' notes are valuable for providing documentation of the patient's mental status upon admission and throughout hospitalization. Changes in behavior, attitude and mood, and orientation usually are noted by the nurses days and weeks before the symptoms are noticed and recorded in the physicians' progress notes. A family history, with emphasis on behavioral difficulties during previous admissions, drug reactions, and mental status changes prior to the current hospitalization is vital.

The electroencephalogram (EEG) should be used routinely in all delirious patients. It adds objectivity to the examination, can confirm the diagnosis, and may provide evidence of neuropathology the physician has not considered, such as complex partial seizures. The usual picture is one of generalized slow waves (θ) in mild delirium, or generalized slowing with intermittent bursts or continuous runs of frontal-central δ-frequencies in more severe conditions. A normal EEG does not rule out delirium. The selective but more frequent use of computerized tomographic (CT) scans or magnetic resonance imaging (MRI) of the brain along with lumbar punctures is also strongly advised.

Examination

Physical examination of the agitated delirious patient is virtually impossible. Thus, the initial approach is simply one of observation. In the more florid conditions, the behavioral manifestations of delirium are unmistakable, and have been listed and discussed above. Much is made about orientation, but many delirious patients, especially in the early stages of the disorder, are fully aware of their surroundings and their situation.

Tests of cognitive functions can be accomplished in a surprising number of delirious patients. Asking the patient to produce a signature is one of the most helpful devices, since handwriting correlates very closely with visuospatial functions. The patient should also be encouraged to write out a sentence, and this material examined for line quality, misuse of words, frequency of spelling errors, and dropped and duplicated letters [18]. The sensitivity of the signature and handwriting to even subtle cerebral changes is impressive and its usefulness in clinical examination cannot be overemphasized.

Other assessments of visuospatial skills, keen indicators of brain function, should also be vigorously attempted. The patient should be asked to draw a circle, square and triangle and, using the circle as a clock face, to set the hands to a specific time. The patient's performance on these tasks is observed for comprehension, concentration, cooperation, pathological anxiety, distractability, and the remembering of instructions. The material is assessed for accuracy of reproduction, line quality, closure of the figures, and organization of the constituent elements of each figure. Errors of reproduction and difficulties with execution are significant for probable cerebral disorder, and frank distortions strengthen the likelihood. The speed with which the task is carried out, especially the setting of time, is a direct measure of cerebral cortical reactivity, and reflects the speed with which the patient is able to process complex information. The venerable subtracting of serial sevens, and asking the patient to spell 'cat' and 'world' backwards are without demonstrable clinical value, as are naming presidents, identifying state capitals, or interpreting proverbs. The Mini Mental Status Examination (MMSE) lacks sufficient sensitivity to even gross neuropathology and should not be relied upon as a screening device. Difficulties in a wider range of cognitive tasks than covered by the MMSE is necessary to establish the diagnosis of delirium. Reliance on a numerical score for the diagnosis of delirium, encouraged by the MMSE, is not only foolhardy, but irresponsible medical practice.

Treatment

The model for managing delirium is similar to one proposed for the treatment of delirium tremens [19]. The method advocates quick and aggressive intervention, giving the majority of the appropriate medication in the early hours of the disorder, with rapid titration to ever-decreasing maintenance levels when the behavioral manifestations of the condition are resolved. Clinical logic suggests that because the offended organ is the brain, with the patient experiencing loss of diurnal rhythm and a prominent sleep disorder which threatens exhaustion, intervention should be aimed at putting both to rest.

Rapid and safe sedation of acutely agitated patients is paramount for several reasons: (1) to prevent injury to themselves or medical personnel; (2) to keep them from disconnecting themselves from life-sustaining equipment or interfering with essential care; (3) to avoid inducing cardiorespiratory instability, and (4) to allow for the prompt investigation of possible reversible causes.

The immediate goal of treatment of the agitated delirious patient is sedation, using the highest doses of drug(s) necessary to quickly and safely accomplish the job. Phenothiazines, because they are potent α-adrenergic blockers, can cause substantial hypotension and therefore have no place in critical care medicine. Diazepam should be avoided because of its long half-life and the risk of drug accumulation with repeated dosing.

The use of the narcotics morphine sulfate or meperidine, both capable of producing delirium, may exacerbate brain failure. In frequently repeated doses, meperidine can cause seizures and death [20]. Because more potent and safer narcotics are available, the use of meperidine should be avoided. Pancuronium (Pavulon)-induced paralysis is not warranted as front-line therapy for delirium. Four-point physical restraints should only be used as a temporary safety measure. Placing a floridly delirious patient in front of a television set or supplying him with a clock and calendar for the purpose of orientation, as is routinely suggested in the literature, is without demonstrated therapeutic value.

The combination of a neuroleptic, benzodiazepine, and narcotic has been found to be the optimal approach to the treatment of delirium [12]. The intravenous (i.v.) route is preferred, because it works faster and obviates the need for repeated intramuscular injections, which further traumatize the patient. Oral dosing, which is recommended in some textbooks, is not usually possible and in fact is inappropriate in this situation. Combination therapy is more effective than single-agent therapy and prevents having to resort to the one-drug megadose approach, with its unknown risks.

Haloperidol (Haldol), lorazepam (Ativan), and hydromorphone (Dilaudid), each the most potent agent in its class, are the drugs of choice. Partiality to this combination stems from observations that together the three medications produce notable results in cases where one drug alone or even two in combination are insufficiently effective.

These three drugs have specific advantages over all other medications, such as short-term half-life, and an absence of clinically important major active metabolites, an important consideration not only in the elderly, but in patients with hepatic and renal impairments. These qualities make them ideal for long-term administration where accumulation kinetics is to be avoided. All have also proved to be safe and efficacious in a wide range of doses.

Clinical experience with hydromorphone, a semisynthetic narcotic, suggests that it may be less of a respiratory depressant than other narcotics and that it is a more potent analgesic than morphine sulfate. Regular administration of a low dose of hydromorphone is warranted, because it is not always possible to determine whether pain may be contributing to a delirious patient's agitation, and because this approach seems to enhance the effects of haloperidol and lorazepam.

Ultimately, experience with the regimen will determine starting doses, but initially, the following approach is suggested. Treatment should be started with 3 mg of haloperidol followed immediately by 0.5 mg each of lorazepam and hydromorphone. The hydromorphone is given on a 3-hourly basis, and the medications are injected intravenously in less than 1 min each, regardless of the doses used.

If, within 20 min, the patient shows little or no response to the first injection, then 5 mg of haloperidol and 0.5–2 mg of lorazepam should be given. Little or no response to this within the next 20 min should be followed by 10 mg of haloperidol and 2–10 mg of lorazepam hourly until the patient is effectively sedated, that is, unresponsive to verbal stimuli but responsive to vigorous flexion-extension movements of the arms. At 10 mg, the haloperidol dose is kept constant, and the lorazepam dose is adjusted to the level of sedation desired.

When the patient is sedated, the lorazepam is discontinued. The dose of haloperidol is reduced by 50%, and the time between administrations is doubled. Hydromorphone, 0.5 mg, is continued every 3 h.

The patient's emergence from sedation and the quality of revival are closely monitored. If emergence is characterized by restlessness, haloperidol and lorazepam should be restarted at the highest effective doses previously used and given every 1–3 h to maintain prolonged sedation for the next 12–18 h. At that time, the above tapering procedure is again followed.

In severe, refractory cases, 240 mg/day of haloperidol and of lorazepam can each be safely given for a number of days. Such doses have been used for 2 weeks without untoward incident [1, 12, 16]. However, less than 100 mg/

day each of haloperidol and of lorazepam are adequate for most cases. Doses above 10 mg/h are generally not required, and in fact confer no additional clinical benefits. Most patients usually respond to treatment within the first 20–30 min, and almost all settle by the end of an hour.

Patient improvement must guide the physician in determining when to discontinue treatment; this decision is highly empirical. Most patients require maintenance therapy once the acute episode has passed, and bedtime dosing with haloperidol (5–10 mg) and lorazepam (0.5–4 mg) for several nights to a week is recommended. The i.v. route can be utilized indefinitely if need be, but oral dosing at this stage of treatment is equally effective. These bedtime doses of haloperidol (5–10 mg i.v.) and lorazepam (0.5–4 mg i.v.) usually suffice for primary treatment of the less florid episodes of delirium, regardless of associated conditions or patient age.

Close monitoring of the amount and quality of the patient's sleep is essential, because disturbed sleep is usually a harbinger of recurrent delirium. In the intensive care unit, where night is seldom allowed to occur, physicians should instruct the nursing staff not to administer bedbaths and other similar nonessential procedures between 9 p.m. and 6 a.m.

This combination drug regimen has proved to be without equal in providing swift, safe, and controllable sedation of even the most severely agitated patient in acute brain failure. This regimen has virtually no effects on cardiac, pulmonary, renal, hepatic, or hematopoietic functions. There are no absolute contraindications, including chemotherapy protocols currently in use, both experimental and approved. Textbook admonitions to the contrary, these medications can be safely used even in hypothyroidism [16]. With high doses of haloperidol, in this combination or even alone, extrapyramidal symptoms are rare [16, 21, 22].

The i.v. use of haloperidol, which is finding increasing favor in medicine, is not approved by the FDA. Therefore, clinicians should obtain permission to use this route through the appropriate hospital committee.

The physician treating delirium must be guided by several important principles. Delirium is a medical emergency, and drug therapy of the condition is a major somatic procedure. During the induction phase, the constant bedside attendance of a physician experienced in the diagnosis and treatment of the condition, supported by a knowledgeable medical nursing staff, is required. Delirious patients can be safely treated with this protocol on general medical and surgical wards if appropriate clinical safeguards are observed. However, transfer to the intensive care unit is advised if prolonged sedation is required.

'As needed' (prn) orders have no place in the treatment of delirious patients. Decisions about dosages and schedules should be made by a physician experienced in the use of the required drugs.

While delirium is undeniably a dangerous neurological disorder, it is also a humanly painful experience in the extreme. Many patients feel tremendously embarrassed and ashamed by their behavior and after they have recovered are loath to bring the matter up on their own.

The management of delirium, therefore, is not complete without informing the patient and his family of the diagnosis, and stressing to them that the bizarre behavior has no deep psychological significance, and is involuntary. No matter how out of control the patient may be, he should be reassured that his condition is medical, is probably temporary, that the medical and nursing staff will protect him from harm, and that medications will be used to palliate the extreme nature of his terrifying condition. Frequent reassurances at the time of examination, and after the episode has abated and remitted, are important features of comprehensive care of the delirious cancer patient.

References

1 Adams, F.: Neuropsychiatric evaluation and treatment of delirium in the critically ill cancer patient. Cancer Bull. *36:* 156–160 (1984).

2 Engel, G.; Romano, J.: Delirium a syndrome of cerebral insufficiency. Chron. Dis. *9:* 260–277 (1959).

3 Adams, F.; Larson, D.; Goepfert, H.: Does the diagnosis of depression in head and neck cancer mask organic brain disease? Otolaryngol. Head Neck Surg. *92:* 618–624 (1984).

4 Davis, B.; Fernandez, F.; Adams, F.; Holmes, V.; Levy, J.; Lewis, D.; Neidhart, J.: Diagnosis of dementia in cancer patients. Psychosomatics *28* (1987).

5 Young, D.F.; Posner, J.B.: Nervous system toxiciy of the chemotherapeutic agents. Handbook of clinical neurology, vol. 39, pp. 91–129 (North-Holland, Amsterdam 1980).

6 Henson, R.A.; Urich, H.: Cancer and the nervous system: the neurological manifestations of systemic malignant disease (Blackwell, Oxford 1982).

7 Lipowski, Z.J.: Delirium updated. Compreh. Psychiat. *21:* 190–196 (1980).

8 Lipowski, Z.J.: Delirium (acute confusional state); in Vinken, Bruyn, Klawans, Handbook of clinical neurology, vol. 2(46), pp. 523–559 (Elsevier, New York 1985).

9 Lipowski, Z.J.: Delirium. Acute brain failure in man, pp. 152–197 (Thomas, Springfield 1980).

10 Lipowski, Z.J.: Transient cognitive disorders (delirium, acute confusional states) in the elderly. Am. J. Psychiat. *140:* 1426–1436 (1983).

11 Freemon, F.R.: Organic mental disease, pp. 81–94 (SP Medical & Scientific Books, New York 1981).

12 Adams, F.: Delirium: an optimal treatment approach. Hosp. Ther. *1987:* 29–42.
13 Shapiro, J.M.; Westphal, L.M.; White, P.F.; et al.: Midazolam infusion for sedation in the intensive care unit: effect on adrenal function. Anesthesiology *64:* 394–398 (1986).
14 White, P.F.: Personal communication.
15 Plum, F.; Posner, J.B.: The pathologic physiology of signs and symptoms of coma. The diagnosis of stupor and coma; 3rd ed., pp. 1–86 (David, Philadelphia 1982).
16 Adams, F.; Fernandez, F.; Andersson, B.: Emergency pharmacotherapy of delirium in the critically ill cancer patient. Psychosomatics *27:* suppl., pp. 33–38 (1986).
17 Massie, M.J.; Holland, J.; Glass, E.: Delirium in terminally ill cancer patients. Am. J. Psychiat. *140:* 1048–1050 (1983).
18 Chedru, F.; Geschwind, N.: Writing disturbances in acute confusional states. Neuropsychologia *10:* 343–353 (1972).
19 Sellers, E.M.; Kalant, H.: Alcohol intoxication withdrawal. New Engl. J. Med. *294:* 757–762 (1976).
20 Kaiko, R.F.; Foley, K.M.; Grabinski, P.Y.; et al.: Central nervous system excitatory effects of meperidine in cancer patients. Ann. Neurol. *13:* 180–185 (1983).
21 Tesar, G.; Murray, G.; Cassem, N.H.: Use of high-dose intravenous haloperidol in the treatment of agitated cardiac patients. J. clin. Psychopharmacol. *5:* 344–347 (1985).
22 Cassem, N.H.: Critical care psychiatry; in Shoemaker, Thompson, Critical care: state of the art, vol. 4, pp. D1–31 (Society of Critical Care Medicine, Fullerton 1983).

Frank Adams, MD, FRCPC, Division of Neuropsychiatric Oncology, Neurobehavioral Center and Pain Service, The Ontario Cancer Institute, The Princess Margaret Hospital, Toronto M4X 1K9 (Canada)

Adv. psychosom. Med., vol. 18, pp. 37–53 (Karger, Basel 1988)

Understanding Denial in Cancer Patients

Margaret S. Wool

Department of Psychiatry, Rhode Island Hospital, Providence, R.I., USA

Introduction

Denial is recognized as an important mechanism in a number of medical and psychiatric illnesses. In some conditions denial is identified as an integral feature of the condition. Examples of those illnesses include anorexia nervosa, alcoholism, and psychosis. In others, such as life-threatening illness, denial is not part of the condition per se, but is involved in the process of emotional adjustment to the disease [McKendry and Logan, 1982; Shaw et al., 1985; Coelho et al., 1974; Peck, 1972; Schoenberg et al., 1974]. Denial varies in its severity, persistence, and pervasiveness [Weisman, 1972]; yielding a broad range of clinical manifestations and effects on adaptive functioning [Lazarus, 1983]. What do these different manifestations look like clinically? How can the adaptive value or liability of this defense mechanism be evaluated? What interventions are useful when cancer patients exhibit denial? The answers to these questions will be addressed in the pages to follow.

Definitions of Denial

The defense mechanism denial is understood as the unconscious disavowal or negation of a perceived external threat [Freud, 1966]. The German translation of denial is 'Leugnung', which means 'it has not happened' [Sandler, 1985, pp. 528–529]. When faced with sudden overwhelming loss, as in bereavement, a common first reaction is denial [Lindemann, 1944]. Kubler-Ross [1969] identified denial at a similar point for cancer patients. Upon first learning a cancer diagnosis, many patients cannot accept the news and, for a time at least, deny it. These two examples involve manifestations of denial that are severe and pervasive, but usually fairly short-lived. Most individuals do come to terms with crisis and loss by gradually acknowledging and accepting painful realizations. Since the capacity to 'test reality', or accurately perceive the world, is an indicator of mental health, individuals who exhibit transient denial are not considered mentally ill.

Another common form of denial is what could be called normal denial — the denial of everyday life which aids our capacity to cope with stress. In contrast to the above examples of denial of sudden stress or crisis, 'normal' denial is not severe or pervasive. It is a negation of dangers of daily life which permits optimal functioning without a crippling sense of anxiety. Most people do not constantly think of the risk of accident while traveling, though some risk is present. To do so would probably impair one's capacity to operate a vehicle safely.

The view of denial as a pathological defense mechanism is based upon the observation of individuals whose use of denial is severe, pervasive, and persistent.

> The infantile ego resorts to denial in order not to become aware of some painful impression from without... The denial of reality is completed and confirmed when in his fantasies, words or behavior, the child reverses the facts [Freud, 1966, p. 89].

While denial is considered a normal mechanism in children, a more mature individual should have developed a broader repertoire of defenses which shield the ego from anxiety while permitting adequate reality testing.

> The organization of the mature ego becomes unified through synthesis and this method of denial is then discarded and is resumed only if the relation to reality has been gravely disturbed and the function of reality testing suspended [Freud, 1966, p. 90].

The damage to reality testing that accompanies persistent and severe denial has led mental health clinicians to classify it as a 'primitive' defense. When defense mechanisms are ordered in a developmental hierarchy, denial is placed along with projection at the lower end of the spectrum, associated with psychosis [Vaillant, 1971].

'Extreme denial' is a term applied to individuals whose denial of their symptoms or aspects of their illness is so pervasive and persistent that it may jeopardize aspects of their physical well-being, intimate social attachments, and ultimate prognosis. In these cases, the defense mechanism does not appear to serve the patient's overall adaptation, though immediate anxiety may be mitigated. Rather, extreme denial interferes with responses that would facilitate the seeking of health care and appropriate medical treatment [Wool, 1986; Wool and Goldberg, 1986]. In one study of cancer patients, 'Eight percent of [the] population avoided medical help until they could no longer operate independently. Only when they were unable to care for themselves did they yield to family or community pressure' [Hackett et al.,

1973, p. 18]. Patients labeled extreme deniers exhibit inhibition in responding to bodily changes by mobilizing timely help-seeking behaviors.

Among the commonly accepted uses of the word 'denial' are expressions of denial in everyday life, as a response to a life crisis and as a maladaptive and pathological response to a life crisis. These different uses encompass a wide range of adaptive functioning from normal to pathological. It is because of this lack of specificity in the use of the word denial that clinicians must think in terms of a 'differential diagnosis' of denial.

The foregoing descriptions are intended to convey some of the broad range of variation in possible manifestations of denial. The implications for research and clinical practice of these different expressions of denial are significant. Clinical intervention, as will be discussed later, must be guided by an assessment of the specific nature of denial: its severity, persistence, and effect on coping. Empirical studies may reveal different findings, in part, as a result of different manifestations of denial. 'As a social strategy, denying depends on what is being denied, and when, how, and to whom the denial is expressed' [Weisman, 1986, p. 61].

Research Contributions

Studies of Denial in Medical Patients

As noted above, denial is recognized as playing a role in the process of adaptation to many forms of trauma or crisis. The adjustment to acute or chronic medical illness is no exception [Rosen, 1950; Thomas, et al., 1983] and has been the subject of empirical investigation. In patients with polycystic kidney disease denial has been found to be associated with disruption in communication, social support, and appropriate health-related behaviors [Manjoney and McKegney, 1978–79]. Manjoney and McKegney [1978–79] cite other studies finding denial to be adaptive in dialysis patients. A study of asthmatic patients found that those who denied or minimized response to their symptoms had a higher rate of rehospitalization than patients who were vigilant and reported anxiety. Vigilant patients were more likely to act promptly when warning signs developed, and hence obtained treatment in less acute states. Patients who denied the severity or implications of symptoms were slower to take health-oriented measures, and more often required emergency hospital admission [Lazarus, 1983].

In patients suffering from acute myocardial infarction, the presence and influence of denial has received considerable attention in the literature

[Prince et al., 1982; Levenson et al., 1984]. In some instances denial appears to be associated with increased survival [Hackett and Cassem, 1974], while in other cases, rehabilitation is compromised when denial interferes with recognition of the need to change behavior and life-style [Soloff, 1977–78; Dimsdale and Hackett, 1982]. Shaw et al. [1985] studied 30 patients with documented myocardial infarction. Measuring denial according to Hackett and Cassem's [1974] interview format, they found no differences in severity of illness or incidence of complications in 6-month follow-up based upon variation in level of denial. The study also revealed that deniers acquired significantly less information about their physical condition. Beisser [1979] referred to a related study which found more post-surgical complications in deniers than nondeniers.

The contradictory nature of the findings of these various studies have yet to be resolved. Several factors which have relevance to the apparent disagreement are differences in operational definitions of denial, and determination of its duration, pervasiveness and context. The timing of the assessment of denial is also an important factor. Since denial is viewed as a normal initial response, it is likely to be more prevalent when subjects are interviewed immediately following a traumatic event, such as diagnosis or surgery. Presence of significant denial substantially later in the course of an illness is likely to reflect a different and less adaptive coping process.

The Use of Denial Among Cancer Patients

Similar to the research with cardiac patients, the use of denial among cancer patients has been recognized as complex and having varying effects on the process of adaptation. Bahnson and Bahnson [1969] asserted that 'repressive ego defenses are the most outstanding and characteristic features' among cancer patients (554). In some cases denial appears to reduce anxiety and promote optimal functioning under stress, while in others denial is associated with excessive delay in help-seeking and poor compliance with medical treatment [Pfefferbaum et al., 1977–78; Schoenberg, 1979; Levine and Zigler, 1975; Schmale, 1976; Kagen, 1976].

Certain nodal points in the illness experience are thought to trigger heightened defensive reactions. These include diagnosis, recurrence, termination of treatment, and deaths of other familiar patients [Gorzynski and Massie, 1981]. In light of these observations, the timing of an assessment of the presence of denial is a very relevant problem.

Weisman [1976] studied 163 newly diagnosed cancer patients to understand factors related to emotional vulnerability. Upon analyzing the clinical interview material, Weisman found some form of denial in 47% of the sample during the 6-month period of investigation. In most cases the denial was transient. Among the factors suggesting emotional vulnerability, denial was found to be correlated with the variables of helplessness and apathy. When all 13 vulnerability items were considered, denial was not found to be significantly correlated with vulnerability. This may be a reflection of the complex nature of denial, and the fact that it is employed in ways that can be either adaptive and aid-effective coping or as a maladaptive response to emotional vulnerability.

Methodological Problems with Research on Denial

Some criticisms of earlier studies have been focused upon the use of the label 'denier' in the absence of sufficient interview or follow-up information. Cousins [1982], for example, cited a case in which a woman was labeled as a denier when she refused the recommended mastectomy for a breast tumor. Upon further inquiry he learned that the woman had obtained a second opinion without informing her first doctor. She accepted a lumpectomy from the second physician. Labeling this patient a 'denier' is incorrect. As Dansak and Cordes [1978–79] point out, such terminology should not be based on limited observation of circumscribed behavior without direct and thorough discussion with the patient.

Another criticism of studies of denial in medical patients has been the exclusive focus on denial of illness and lack of attention to more positive aspects of affirmation of health in coping behavior [Beisser, 1979]. Considering coping behavior in terms of a matrix comprising denial and affirmation of health and illness, Beisser believes that self-actualizing behaviors can be more readily appreciated. Thus, this model advocates supporting morale and acceptance of necessary treatments without viewing expressions of hope and optimism as signs of avoidance, denial, or pathology.

In reviewing research findings, one may ask whether deniers are also denying negative feelings, such as alienation, dysphoria, and other variables thought to mark emotional vulnerability. Dimsdale and Hackett [1982] found high denial to be associated with low emotional distress and more advanced cardiac disease. Dimsdale and Hackett's findings suggest that deniers may tend to minimize reporting of dysphoric affect. The tendency to minimize reports of dysphoric feelings would be likely to be manifest in patients' responses to psychological instruments. Thus, when items on a psychological instrument inquire directly about lowered mood state, deniers could be expected to minimize reports of dysphoria. In this way, the face validity of some psychological measures introduces certain obvious problems when trying to evaluate the benefits of denial in coping with serious illnesses. Researchers may assume that denial is associated with less mood disturbance rather than considering the possibility that patients who deny the seriousness of their illness may also deny negative emotions.

In summary, research on denial is troubled with several methodological problems. A primary problem is the lack of consistency in how denial is defined and operationalized. Weisman [1976] is one of the few investigators to distinguish levels of severity and persistence of denial. Since denial is known to be exhibited in different forms, a more refined nosology seems necessary when linking denial to coping and adaptation.

'Diagnosis' of Denial

Denial is a complex and multifaceted phenomenon. Measurement and identification of denial are also complex, and have not been carried out in a uniform fashion in the literature which deals with adjustment to cancer. In a research context, outlining types of denial permits a more precise examination of the manifestations of denial. While the stereotypic case of denial is transient denial of diagnosis, not all patients manifest denial in this form. The issue of varied manifestations of denial is relevant for clinical and for research purposes. Therefore, the clinical manifestations of denial will be described more fully below.

Several authors have developed approaches for classifying types of denial, in the interest of refining the concepts and communication regarding this complex mechanism. Freud referred to denial in fantasy, word and act [Freud, 1966; Sandler, 1985]. Denial in fantasy is the most benign of these three categories. It is inherent in childrens' play, and could also be characterized as daydreaming in both children and adults.

Denial in word and deed bring an intrapsychic event into an interpersonal realm through behavioral expression. Carried into action, denial brings the risk of harm through inadequate response to the demands of reality. In the area of cancer, the act of denial results in unconscious negation of symptoms of illness and, therefore, a disruption of the help-seeking response. This produces a far more serious consequence than the wish-fulfilling fantasy which does not affect behavior. 'Denial is not all bad, nor is affirmation all good. But denial of any problem and therefore of any need to cope correctly sows seeds of dismay and disaster' [Weisman, 1986, p. 75].

Weisman [1972] distinguishes the *fact* of denial from the *process* of denial. The process of denial includes repudiation of some meaningful aspect of reality, and replacement of the repudiated perception with a preferred view or belief. Denial may be focused upon facts, implications of illness, or impending death; labeled as first-, second-, and third-order denial.

Noting the fact of denial fails to describe the meaning of denial for a given individual. One must be able to answer the following questions to give a thorough characterization of an individual's expression of denial: 'What form does the denial take? To whom is the denial communicated? What are the circumstances in which denial is expressed? What is threatened?' [Weisman, 1972, p. 63].

Denial may be directed toward some aspects of the illness experience while realistic assessment of other dimensions is preserved. For example, one 75-year-old patient could cite the exact date of her mastectomy, yet not whether she'd been aware of symptoms the previous summer. Similarly, she was accurate in reporting on the series of tests she had undergone, and which ones revealed favorable findings, yet she could not name the disease which was being investigated. Physical manifestations of the illness may be denied, as in the following case example:

Mr. A., a 78-year-old male patient stated he'd bumped his shoulder 12–20 years prior to presentation. The 'bump' grew progressively and bled. Mr. A. began sleeping with a shirt on and eventually began sleeping on a sofa in the basement. He resisted his family's urging to seek health care until they finally had him removed from the basement by calling a rescue squad. Diagnosis was basal cell epithelioma, which had progressed to the point that his spine was exposed and his hemoglobin subnormal. Delay was explained as related to fear of surgery. Mr. A. had no significant formal medical or psychiatric history, and was compliant once treatment began. In this case, what would have been a simple office curettage required considerable hospitalization and radiation therapy.

Similarly, denial may focus on diagnosis, implications of illness, and/or affective response to the experience of cancer [Wool and Goldberg, 1986].

Denial of Diagnosis. Mr. B. stated that he never had been told what his medical problem was and why he was receiving radiotherapy treatment. We met together with the doctor, where the patient repeated his sense of confusion about the cause of the pain in his chest. The doctor explained the nature of the disease in his lung and his treatment, using the word cancer, and then asked the patient for his understanding of what had just been reviewed. Mr. B. said, 'I don't know, I just have this pain.'

Denial of Implications of Illness. Miss D., a 61-year-old single woman with breast cancer, delayed seeking treatment for seven years though she reported conscious awareness of a lump. She said she knew the lump meant cancer and wasn't surprised by the diagnosis. She said she tried to ignore the growth and eventually applied dressings which helped her 'ignore' it. She stated, 'I watched it. It got bigger and bigger. When it got to the point where I didn't want to look at it, then I put covering on it. Then, under the bra you don't feel anything, you don't see anything... so it's not there anymore.' She finally sought medical attention in the emergency department when she began to hemorrhage. Striking in this woman's history was a mother who died of breast cancer and who exhibited the same aspect of denial and delay.

Some individuals demonstrate simultaneous or rapidly fluctuating denial and awareness, called 'middle knowledge' [Weisman, 1972, p. 65]. While we cannot yet link particular types of denial with specific patient personality types, it might be suggested that variations in the personal experience of emotional threat could influence the expression of this defense. Since denial is seen as an indicator of severe psychopathology, one hypothesis links the presence of extreme denial with immature ego development. Although this area of inquiry has not been studied extensively, the author's recent investigation revealed findings suggestive of support for the above hypothesis [Wool, 1986].

In the field of sociology 'strategies' of denial in cancer patients have been described. Glaser and Strauss [1965, pp. 132–134] noted communication blocks to prevent recognition of facts about the illness, 'juggling time' to cling to an unrealistic but wished for length of survival, and 'comparative references', in which patients compare their condition with other exceptional and favorable cases to gauge their own status.

Finally, McKendry and Logan [1982] designated 'independent', 'dependent', and 'healthy' deniers whose styles of adaptation lead to problems at different phases of the illness. The authors recommend alternate strategies for the management of each type of denier. A nonconfrontational style was suggested for the aggressive independent denier, direct and assertive approaches with the passive dependent denier, and facilitating the healthy denier in the process of resolution.

Establishing the Presence of Denial

Several basic considerations are relevant for assessing a patient's behavior as possibly being denial. A complete biopsychosocial evaluation is the foundation for this assessment [Wallace et al., 1984]. The clinician must screen for serious cognitive impairment which may interfere with patients' capacities to absorb, process, or communicate about their illness. For example, dysphasia from a cerebral metastasis should not be considered denial. Patients with an active major psychiatric disorder, such as schizophrenia, or patients with memory impairment from alcoholism should not be misidentified simply as deniers. Appropriate medical or psychiatric evaluation and treatment should be provided before conclusive assessment of defensive functioning can proceed in a meaningful fashion [Goldberg, 1983].

After assessing the patient for an organic mental disorder or major psychiatric disorder, it is important as the next step to establish what the patient knows. It is clear that one cannot deny a diagnosis that has not first been presented. When many doctors are involved and one has not been identified as the primary coordinator, communication to the patient may become confused or incomplete. At times, this may reflect staff difficulty in approaching the patient directly to discuss the illness. As far as the patient is concerned, however, ignorance cannot be called denial. It is always important to inquire about knowledge of diagnosis. The clinician may accomplish this without introducing the word 'cancer' by asking, 'What is your understanding of why you are in the hospital?', 'What has your doctor told you about your illness?' and other similarly nonthreatening questions [Goldberg and Tull, 1983]. The patient's ability to be direct and accurate in his response to this question will reveal a great deal about his or her comfort with (or need to defend against) the information. A practical technique to prevent confusing denial with communication problems is documentation in the patient's record of what the patient has been told about his disease.

Mechanisms that Masquerade as Denial

Denial cannot be established simply by the fact that patients do not spontaneously talk about their condition. Behaviorally avoidance, suppression, and denial can look alike [Lazarus, 1983]. The distinction between denial and suppression in cancer patients must be determined through the use of careful clinical assessment [Dansak and Cordes, 1978–79]. Suppression is defined as a conscious or semiconscious process in which the defense is directed toward an intrapsychic event, e.g. conflict or impulse. This mechanism is in contrast to denial, which is unconscious and aimed against external threat or internal threat in the form of an intolerable idea. One cannot infer denial when a person simply does not volunteer information about his illness. A better understanding of signs of the patient's unconscious process is required before this designation may be made.

Avoidance represents a knowing effort to shun any circumstances that bring stressful material to the forefront. The individual may know full well that he has cancer, and may feel better able to control his emotional reactions by deflecting conversation away from the topic of his illness. If the behavior were pointed out, the individual would be able to consciously acknowledge it. In marked contrast to denial, patients manifesting avoidance may often experience strong affects, such as anxiety or depression. A contradiction between someone's verbal content and affect may reveal an understanding of the illness that is not being directly expressed. For example, a patient may have a trembling voice or look tearful while saying there is nothing to worry about. In such cases, the individual is likely to be masking a sense of vulnerability with feigned optimism.

Social and Interpersonal Factors

The interpersonal context of the patient with presumed denial must always be considered, since social forces influence a patient's expressed awareness of attitudes toward and behaviors relating to his disease [Mastrovitro, 1974; Silberfarb, 1977–78; Weisman, 1972, 1986; Glaser and Strauss, 1965; Thomas et al., 1983]. Patients respond to subtle social cues of the doctors, caregivers, friends and relatives, and behave in ways that will maximize the sense of support. Patients may also attempt to reduce the emotional burden on family and friends by expressing false hopes. Behaviors designed to increase social support may include avoiding recognition of medical symptoms or the implications of the diagnosis. The social factors noted above are relevant in planning the setting for a clinical interview. For example, seeing the patient alone or with family present may elicit very different responses.

In some families, the threatened loss of a member is so intolerable that denial cannot be relinquished. These families would be characterized generally as maintaining symbiotic, overly dependent, 'enmeshed' attachments or as 'crisis-ridden' [Wallace et al., 1984]. In these cases it may be necessary for a clinician to continue to provide support over an extended period of time. Often a crisis intervention model is useful, involving therapeutic family meetings at times of crisis in the illness such as recurrence or withdrawal of curative therapies [Mor et al., 1987]. 'Going along with the defenses' is a technique which often proves facilitative [Love and Mayer, 1959]. This is an ego-supportive approach in which defenses are not directly challenged, and the family can be helped to relinquish overly defensive coping styles.

An additional formulation for understanding the social dimensions of denial is a contribution from social psychology. The common assumption in the field of psychiatry has been that denial is a barrier to resolution of emotional problems, and would be seen, in the present context, as an obstacle to adjustment to cancer. A sociological perspective suggests that the rejection of a stigmatizing label such as 'mental patient' or 'cancer patient' can be beneficial [O'Mahony, 1982]. A study of denial of mental illness found that:

> The patients who actively rejected identification of the self with the stereotype of the mentally ill were not passive victims of, or collaborators in, an insiduous social labelling process. On the other hand, they did not resort to thoroughgoing or pathological denial of reality in order to distance themselves from the mentally ill. Rather they emphasized their own uniqueness at a time when it was particularly threatened [O'Mahony, 1982, p. 117].

The above formulation of denial as a normal and socially beneficial process has not been studied in cancer patients. Since mental patients and cancer patients both represent stigmatized groups in our culture, O'Mahony's theory presents interesting possibilities for future research in psychosocial oncology.

Refusal of Treatment

It should be pointed out that the refusal of a recommended treatment may nor may not reflect the presence of denial. Certain barriers to accepting treatment are not always legitimate reasons for refusal.Barriers to accepting treatment may include intrapsychic and interpersonal problems, psychiatric disorders, and communications problems with the medical team. These should be viewed as problems to be solved, not legitimate reasons for refusal. On the other hand, some patients may make a considered and deliberate choice to refuse or discontinue medical intervention. With careful review of the patient's and family's knowledge, intention, and other possible medical, psychiatric and communication complications, the refusal may be very legitimate and appropriately accepted. We do a disservice to patients by jumping to the incorrect assumption that refusal or noncompliance is, in itself, an indication of denial [Goldberg, 1983; Roth et al., 1982].

Clinical Implications

The importance of distinguishing denial from other mechanisms is relevant to the following clinical issues. Given the hierarchical formulation of defense mechanisms [Freud, 1966; Vaillant, 1971], patients with extreme manifestations of denial could be assumed to represent a group with relatively immature ego capacities. Intervention strategies, therefore, would need to be tailored to a lower developmental level than for a more mature patient

[Horner, 1979]. Since higher level defenses are, by definition, less pervasive and rigid than primitive ones, those mechanisms which masquerade as denial would be far more accessible to reduction through clinical intervention than is denial. More precise identification of defensive processes can aid in the choice of appropriate treatment strategies [Blanck and Blanck, 1974].

Assessing the Adaptive Effects of Denial

Rather than regarding denial as an undifferentiated phenomenon, identifying the specific aspects of denial that are present lays the groundwork for understanding its potential adaptive or maladaptive effects. This understanding, in turn, helps direct intervention strategies.

The first important question is whether the denial is affecting help-seeking behavior and compliance. The adaptive function depends on the type and magnitude of denial. In some instances, denial helps modulate emotional reactions to the stress of life-threatening illness and eases the patient's course while in treatment. Often, initial denial is replaced by integration of knowledge about the illness, and the adoption of more flexible coping strategies. Since help-seeking and compliance with a medical regimen often represent the most active behaviors to promote one's well-being and survival, persistent, extreme denial and delay threaten prognosis and are considered maladaptive.

A second question is whether the denial is reducing emotional distress. While denial may be adaptive by reducing distress, it can be maladaptive in two extreme situations: the first example would be one in which, due to the absence of anxiety, the patient does not act to obtain help. The other is one in which pervasive denial shields a fragile patient. The extreme denial of diagnosis or illness implications precludes assimilation of medical information. When the disease progresses to the point that it can no longer be ignored, or when participation in treatment requires confrontation by caregivers, denial may fail. When this occurs the patient may feel flooded and may experience a reactive psychosis [Soloff, 1977–78]. In these instances, psychiatric management is indicated. If the patient is not psychotic, signs of depression or anxiety may represent denial functioning maladaptively [Goldberg, 1981].

A successful defense serves to reduce stress and facilitate adjustment. Patients in distress may require a supportive intervention, either directly with the patient or with significant others to foster support [Goldberg and Wool, 1985].

Guidelines for Therapeutic Intervention

The principal aspects of adaptive functioning focused on in work with cancer patients are emotional stability, social support, and compliance with necessary medical treatment. Explicit acknowledgment of diagnosis is really secondary to these broader issues. In attempting to modify extreme denial, the actual goal may be compliance with treatment or reduction of emotional distress, not necessarily the ability to say, 'I have terminal cancer'. With clear goals in mind, an approach which limits the likelihood of anxiety is most likely to be successful.

> 'While anxiety arousal is undoubtedly necessary, there should be a considerably increased effort to introduce new messages which underscore the responsibility of the individual to guard his health for the sake of his family and other significant roles he holds in the community. In addition, accentuated importance should be given to portraying patient-physician relationships as involving cooperation and mutual trust rather than subordination' [Fisher, 1967, p. 678].

Emphasizing to the patient the dire medical consequences of noncompliance would likely lead to intensification of denial and possibly flight. Since the denial is employed to mitigate emotional distress and fear of loss of control, statements less likely to be experienced as threatening are desirable. One might support the idea that trips to the hospital for cancer treatment are inconvenient, but emphasize the family's willingness to accompany the patient. Offering the patient a reasonable choice of appointment times may foster a sense of active involvement and control. In addition, the assignment to a particular staff member may enhance the focus on a relationship rather than a feared medical procedure when anticipating hospital appointments. Specification of the type of denial present and its adaptive or maladaptive functions aid in the decision to try to reduce or modify denial. Practically, if there is low emotional distress and good compliance, a psychotherapy intervention is probably not indicated. If either high emotional distress or poor compliance are present, some intervention should probably be considered. Ego support must accompany gradual confrontation for positive results. One article reported a patient experiencing a psychotic break in response to confrontive intervention. Soloff [1977–78] reported that failure of denial in a post-infarction patient produced a transient psychosis characterized by paranoid ideation and a clear sensorium. Psychiatric consultation and possibly psychotropic medications followed by brief supportive psychotherapy is often indicated in these instances.

When intervention seems indicated, it is important to differentiate support from reassurance. When a patient expresses distress, the listener has several options. Reassurance, saying that things are not so bad, and efforts to cheer the patient up, are often experienced as nonsupportive and communicate the listener's not wanting to be exposed to the patient's emotional pain. When the patient is declining, having someone tolerate this fear, uncertainty, anger, and discomfort with the patient is most therapeutic. It can give the patient courage to be more open with his family and friends, being less fearful that the illness and discomfort will repel needed support. Some families may need professional assistance to improve communication skills.

In many cultures, men are expected to be 'strong' and not show their feelings. Similarly, difficulty with the role transition from breadwinner or homemaker to patient may be associated with guilt and may lead to behaviors that appear to represent denial but actually comprise avoidance of affects that accompany the illness experience. Sensitive discussion with patients of ways in which the disease or treatment has led to disruption of family life-style can help the patient identify issues associated with guilt. By experiencing support from the clinician, the patient may be better able to tolerate painful affect, and improve communication in important relationships. Seeing that shifts in roles can be talked about and accommodated in the family may help diminish the guilt that has led to avoidance and impaired capacity to relate more fully in other interpersonal relationships.

The tone of the interview is more crucial than what specific words are said. Experienced clinicians find that they can talk about almost anything with a patient in an atmosphere of privacy, respect, and comfort. Common taboo subjects are death and sexuality. Not surprisingly, these are often areas of greatest concern to patients and their family members. Techniques which facilitate discussion of these topics include gradual introduction. One would not begin with death or terminal status, for example, but might join the patient in reviewing the history of the illness: what was first noticed, how it was decided to seek medical attention, how the family has reacted, etc. Then it is possible to move gradually into how things are going now, how the family has readjusted, the patient's understanding of the recent decision to discontinue chemotherapy, the fact that his disease has not responded to treatment and his functional status continues to decline. In this way, the clinician shares some of the history with the patient and the momentum of the interview makes discussion of the expected death part of a natural process.

A similar approach would be used to discuss sexual concerns of cancer patients. One might discuss the relationship with the spouse in general and then talk about intimate aspects of the relationship including physical closeness and sexuality. Alternatively, changes in self-esteem and body image as a result of illness or surgery might be important forerunners to a discussion about sexual functioning. The clinician's willingness to gently pursue sensitive material with comfort is often the most persuasive factor in encouraging the patient to do so.

Conclusions

Denial is a way to cope with threat and loss. In individuals with robust emotional resources denial, if needed at all, is usually employed only transiently. It represents a way that people 'buy time' to prepare to assimilate some particularly painful realization, so as not to feel too overwhelmed. In apparently less resilient individuals, more extreme and persistent denial may be evident. When present to a significant degree, denial interferes with recognition of the seriousness of symptoms or implications of illness. The failure to acknowledge important features of the illness can lead to poor health-related behaviors and may have serious medical consequences.

In and of itself, denial is neither good nor bad. The way in which it may assist or impede an individual's adjustment to cancer is the central concern for the oncology clinician. This chapter has reviewed different research findings regarding the use of denial, described various clinical manifestations of the defense, and recommended clinical strategies for assessment and intervention with patients exhibiting denial-like mechanisms.

References

Bahnson, M.B.; Bahnson, C.B.: Ego defenses in cancer patients. Ann. N.Y. Acad. Sci. *164:* 83–96 (1969).

Beisser, A.R.: Denial and affirmation in illness and health. Am. J. Psychiat. *136:* 1026–1030 (1979).

Blanck, G.; Blanck, R.: Ego psychology theory and practice (Columbia University Press, New York 1974).

Coehlo, G.; Hamburg, D.; Adams, J.: Coping and adaptation (Basic Books, New York 1974).

Cousins, N.: Denial: Are sharper definitions needed? J. Am. med. Ass. *284:* 210–212 (1982).

Dansak, D.; Cordes, R.: Cancer: Denial or suppression? Int. J. Psychiat. Med. *9:* 257–262 (1978–79).

Dimsdale, J.E.; Hackett, T.P.: Effect of denial on cardiac health and psychological assessment. Am. J. Psychiat. *139:* 1477–1480 (1982).
Fisher, S.: Motivation for patient delay. Archs gen. Psychiat. *16:* 676–678 (1967).
Freud, A.: The ego and the mechanisms of defense (Hogarth, London 1966).
Glaser, B.; Strauss, A.: Awareness of dying (Aldine, Chicago 1965).
Goldberg, R.J.: Management of depression in the patient with advanced cancer. J. Am. med. Ass. *246:* 373–376 (1981).
Goldberg, R.J.: Systematic understanding of cancer patients who refuse treatment. Psychother. Psychosom. *39:* 180–189 (1983).
Goldberg, R.J.; Tull, R.M.: The psychosocial dimensions of cancer (Free Press, New York 1983).
Goldberg. R.J.; Wool, M.S.: Psychotherapy for the spouses of lung cancer patients: assessment of an intervention. Psychother. Psychosom. *43:* 141–150 (1985).
Gorzynsky, J.G.; Massie, M.J.: How to manage the depression of cancer. Your Pt. Ca. *8:* 25–30 (1981).
Hackett, T.P.; Cassem, N.H.: Development of a quantitative rating scale to assess denial. J. psychosom. Res. *18:* 93–100 (1974).
Hackett, T.P.; Cassem, N.H.; Raker, J.W.: Patient delay in cancer. New Engl. J. Med. *289:* 14–20 (1973).
Horner, A.J.: Object relations and the developing ego in therapy (Aronson, New York 1979).
Kagen, L.: Use of denial in adolescents with bone cancer. Health S.W. *1:* 71–87 (1976).
Kübler-Ross, E.: On death and dying (Macmillan, New York 1969).
Lazarus, R.S.: The costs and benefits of denial; in Breznitz, The denial of stress (Int. Universities Press, New York 1983).
Levenson, J.L.; Kay, R.; Monteferrante, J.; Herman, M.V.: Denial predicts favorable outcome in unstable angina pectoris. Psychom. Med. *46:* 25–32 (1984).
Levine, J.; Zigler, E.: Denial and self-image in stroke, lung cancer, and heart disease patients. J. consult. clin. Psychol. *43:* 751–757 (1975).
Lindemann, E.: Symptomatology and management of acute grief. Am. J. Psychiat. *101:* 141–149 (1944).
Love, S.; Mayer, H.: Going along with the defenses in resistive families. Social Casework *2:* 69–74 (1959).
Manjoney, D.M.; McKegney, F.P.: Individual and family coping with polycystic kidney disease: the harvest of denial. Int. J. Psychiat. Med. *9:* 19–31 (1978–79).
Mastrovitro, R.C.: Cancer: awareness and denial. Clin. Bull. *4:* 142–146 (1974).
McKendry, M.; Logan, R.L.: The recognition and management of denial in patients after myocardial infarction. Aust. N.Z.J. Med. *12:* 607–611 (1982).
Mor, V.; Guadagnoli, E.; Wool, M.S.: An examination of the concrete service needs of advanced cancer patients. J. psychosoc. Oncology *5(1):* 1–15 (Spring, 1987).
O'Mahony, P.D.: Psychiatric patient denial of mental illness as a normal process. Br. J. med. Psychol. *55:* 109–118 (1982).
Peck, A.: Emotional reactions to having cancer. J. Roentgenol. Radium Ther. nucl. Med. *114:* 591–599 (1972).
Pfefferbaum, B.; Pasnau, R.; Jamison, K.; Wellisch, D.: A comprehensive program of psychosocial care for mastectomy patients. Int. J. Psychiat. Med. *8:* 63–72 (1977–78).
Prince, R.; Frasure-Smith, N.; Rolicz-Woloszyk, E.: Life stress, denial and outcome in ischemic heart disease patients. J. psychosom. Res. *26:* 23–31 (1982).

Rosen, V.H.: The role of denial in acute postoperative affective reactions following removal of body parts. Psychosom. Med. *12:* 356–361 (1950).
Roth, L.H.; Applebaum, P.S.; Sallee, R.; Reynolds, C.F., III; Huber, G.: The dilemma of denial in the assessment of competency to refuse treatment. Am. J. Psychiat. *139:* 910–913 (1982).
Sandler, J.: The analysis of defense: the ego and the mechanisms of defense revisited (Int. Universities Press, New York 1985).
Schmale, A.: Psychological reactions to recurrences, metastases, or disseminated cancer. Int. J. Rad. Biol. rel. Stud. Phys. Med. *1:* 515–520 (1976).
Schoenberg, B.: Sex after mastectomy: counseling husband and wife. Med. Aspects human Sex. *2:* 88–100 (1979).
Schoenberg, B.; Carr, A.C.; Kutscher, A.H.; Peretz, D.; Goldberg, I. (eds): Anticipatory grief (Columbia University Press, New York 1974).
Shaw, R.E.; Cohen, F.; Doyle, B.; Palesky, J.: The impact of denial and repressive style on information gain and rehabilitation outcomes in myocardial infarction patients. Psychosom. Med. *47:* 262–273 (1985).
Silberfarb, P.M.: Psychiatric themes in the rehabilitation of mastectomy patients. Int. J. Psychiat. Med. *8:* 159–167 (1977–78).
Soloff, P.H.: Denial and rehabilitation of the post-infarction patient. Int. J. Psychiat. Med. *8:* 125–132 (1977–78).
Thomas, S.A.; Sappington, E.; Gross, H.S.; Noctor, M.; Friedmann, E.; Lynch, J.J.: Denial in coronary care patients — an objective reassessment. Heart Lung *12:* 74–80 (1983).
Vaillant, G.: Theoretical hierarchy of adaptive ego mechanisms. Archs gen. Psychiat. *2:* 107–118 (1971).
Wallace, S.R.; Goldberg, R.J.; Slaby, A.E.: Clinical social work in health care: new biopsychosocial approaches (Praeger, New York 1984).
Weisman, A.: On dying and denying: a study of psychiatric terminality (Behavioral Publications, New York 1972).
Weisman, A.: Early diagnosis of vulnerability in cancer patients. Am. J. med. Sci. *271:* 187–196 (1976).
Weisman, A.D.: The coping capacity, on the nature of being mortal (Human Sciences Press, New York 1986).
Wool, M.S.: An exploratory study of extreme denial in breast cancer patients; unpubl. doct. diss. (Smith College School for Social Work, Northampton 1986).
Wool, M.S.; Goldberg, R.J.: Assessment of denial in cancer patients: implications for intervention. J. psychosoc. Onc. *4:* 1–14 (1986).

Margaret S. Wool, ACSW, PhD, Department of Psychiatry, Rhode Island Hospital, 593 Eddy Street, Providence, RI 02903 (USA)

Adv. psychosom. Med., vol. 18, pp. 54–65 (Karger, Basel 1988)

Psychotherapy with Cancer Patients

Margaret W. Linn

Social Science Research, Veterans Administration Medical Center,
University of Miami School of Medicine, Miami, Fla., USA

This chapter will review briefly personality and stress factors as these relate to cancer with implications for psychotherapy, psychological reactions to cancer, factors associated with longer survival, psychotherapeutic intervention studies, selection of patients for therapy, and models for psychotherapy.

Personality and Psychological Factors in Cancer

The role of the emotions in the development, onset, and course of cancer has interested those involved in the treatment of the disease for over a century. Studies in the late 1950s and 1960s were concerned largely with psychological factors in the etiology of cancer. Repressed emotional conflicts associated with loss of an important person in the individual's life [1]; patterns of separation, loss, depression, and hopelessness [2]; and inability to express negative emotions, particularly anger, coupled with significant loss [3, 4] were reportedly found in patients with malignant disease. Most of the studies, however, were carried out after individuals had been diagnosed as having cancer, and the possibility that psychological reactions, such as hopelessness, resulted from the individual knowing that he or she had cancer could not be determined.

Although studies after the 1960s focused more on the concomitant emotional problems of cancer patients than on the role of emotions in the etiology of cancer, the idea that a cancer-prone personality exists has not been abandoned. In fact, Temoshok and Fox [5] recently described what may be a type C personality that is associated with cancer proneness. Type Cs work hard at maintaining a pleasant interpersonal atmosphere. They control angry expressions. They want to be welliked and pleasant. They suppress or repress negative emotions, maintain a happy façade, and do not express dysphoric emotions.

In view of the early emphasis on cancer as a psychosomatic disease, precipitated by arrested personality development and emotional distress, it is not surprising that early psychotherapy was focused on patients in whom psychological assessments showed neurotic features [6]. Treatment drew heavily on psychoanalysis and psychoanalytic psychotherapy, popular at that time. Goals were directed toward replacing object losses and finding new outlets for frustrated and sublimated emotions.

Stressful Life Events, Immune Function, and Cancer

Concomitant with the studies of personality characteristics as causative factors in cancer were other studies that also looked at etiological factors but focused on environmental stressors rather than personality in onset of cancer. Major stressful life events were found to be associated with development of a number of diseases including cancer [7, 8]. Interest has increased in the role of stress in cancer as a number of studies have demonstrated a relationship between psychosocial stressors and decreased immune function [9–12]. Stress and decreased immune function has been associated with development and growth of neoplasms in animals [13, 14]. Furthermore, immunosuppression has been reported in depressed patients [15], and the incidence of cancer in depressed individuals has been found to be high [16]. So much interest has been generated in these mind-body connections that a new field of psychoneuroimmunology has emerged. From both animal and human studies, certain factors appear to mediate between stressors and psychophysical reactions and consequences such as disease. Adaptive coping styles, perceived control over stressors, and social support are a few among a number of mediators or modifiers of stress reactions. Such studies have opened the door for new approaches in the psychosocial treatment of cancer patients both in the areas of behavioral medicine as well as in psychotherapy.

Regardless of whether personality characteristics interact with stress in the onset of cancer, the occurrence of cancer itself is a major stressful event. It is also an ongoing stressor in that individuals face debilitating effects from chemotherapy and radiation or mutilating effects of surgery. Even those who cope well with treatment often worry about the possibility of recurrence of cancer or fatal outcomes. Those who have a recurrence may find all of the old stress reactions reactivated and intensified.

Psychological Reactions to Diagnosis of Cancer

Psychological reactions to having cancer include anxiety, anger, decreased self-esteem, and depression. Some cancer patients develop psychiatric conditions. Derogatis et al. [17] reported a 47% prevalence of psychiatric disorders in cancer patients using DSM-III criteria. Over half (68%) were diagnosed as having an adjustment disorder. Rates of depression among cancer patients are also high but vary according to how depression was measured. Self-reported depression in cancer patients ranges from 23% [18] to 74% [19]; however, this undoubtedly includes depressed mood and distress in addition to clinical depression. More rigorously assessed diagnoses, using DSM-III criteria, suggest between 6% [17] and 42% [20] rates of depression. The extent of psychopathology in patients is further associated with stage of disease, physical disability, and morbidity from cancer treatments.

Psychological Factors and Survival from Cancer

Some psychological patterns have been associated with length of survival. Similar to the personality factors that were implicated in onset of cancer, a number of studies found patients who were cooperative and reluctant to express their emotions, particularly negative feelings such as anger, died earlier [21, 22]. More recently, patients who expressed more anxiety, hostility, and alienation — in other words, they expressed their negative emotions — were found to be longer survivors of cancer [23]. Further, breast cancer patients who had a fighting spirit or used denial were found, in another study [24], to have better outcomes than those who stoically accepted cancer or reacted with helplessness or hopelessness.

Psychotherapeutic Interventions

Despite the well-documented psychological distress associated with cancer, not many studies have evaluated the use of psychotherapy for cancer patients, and those that have show conflicting findings. Watson [25] has pointed out some of the limitations of these studies that confound comparisons of results between studies. For example, in some studies it is not clear what is meant by 'cancer patient' in that a large number of the patients may not know their diagnosis and thus not be under the same amount of stress as others who do. Many studies do not have control groups. Types of treatment interventions differ and often are ill defined. The focus for evaluation is usually whether treatment benefits the patients, but assessments and/or statistical comparisons may be inadequate to answer this question.

One way of classifying studies of psychotherapeutic interventions is by group versus individual approaches with early-stage versus late-stage cancer patients.

Group Psychotherapy. Most group interventions have focused on some aspect of social support and/or education. Several studies [26, 27] indicate that social support groups are effective in reducing emotional distress in cancer patients. In one of these studies [27], breast cancer patients randomly assigned to treatment and followed for one year reported less tension, confusion, fatigue, phobias, and maladaptive coping styles than did those assigned to a control group. However, levels of depression were similar in the two groups. Weisman et al. [28] also reported benefits from group therapy in that cancer patients who attended had less distress than did a control group. Within the therapy group, two types of intervention were used and found to be equally effective. One used an experiential model and the other used a more didactic approach coupled with relaxation. Another study [29], however, found no benefits from the same two types of groups in that a psychotherapy group and a relaxation/education group showed similar results. This study, however, did not use a control group for comparison of findings. It is known that support groups are used mostly by white, middle- to upper-class women, thus are limited to a small proportion of cancer patients. In one study [30], men with cancer improved in a group when the group was focused on educational intervention compared with controls. Also, men assigned randomly to a social support or control group, in another study [31], showed no benefit from treatment. Therefore, it would seem that men gain more from an educational rather than support focus.

A few studies have evaluated group therapy for late-stage cancer patients. The study described earlier by Spiegel et al. [27] showed positive results for therapy that was focused on problems of terminal illness, relationships with family and medical staff, and living as fully as possible in the face of death. Another study [32] of group therapy for late-stage breast cancer patients found counselled patients had more confidence in the medical treatment team and greater comfort; however, affective states were not assessed. Obviously, groups are not the answer for every cancer patient that needs treatment. At the same time, groups offer some advantages that make them worth further study. For example, it has been shown that social support can reduce psychological distress during times of stress [33, 34]. Groups that build on provision of education, encouragement of expression of feelings, sharing of experiences, and modeling of coping efficacy should have the potential for benefits to cancer patients.

Individual Treatment. A crises intervention approach to individual therapy for women with gynecological cancers was evaluated by Capone et al. [35]. No clear benefits in mood were found; however, more of the therapy patients returned to premorbid levels of sexual adjustment earlier and reported more increased self-esteem than did matched controls. Similarly, another crises intervention approach to counselling found no differences from a self-help comparison group [36]. Neither group reduced depression in patients. Less distortion of body image was found in both groups compared with controls. Patients with a variety of types of cancer were studied with a multimethod technique that included counselling, environmental manipulation, and education [37]. Treatment was tailored to meet the needs of each patient. Patients receiving therapy had a better outlook on life and returned to work more often than did the comparison group. This study, however, found positive changes in the patients' mood 6 months after discharge from the hospital. Watson [38] described individual counselling for mastectomy patients in which patients were helped to focus on adaptive coping. Compared to a control group, those who received therapy made a more rapid recovery, had less depression, and greater feelings of personal control. Forester et al. [39] found that individual psychotherapy provided to patients receiving radiotherapy improved emotional and physical manifestations of distress as compared with controls who received only radiotherapy. Men seemed to suffer more distress than women but also had a greater response to psychotherapy. Bloom et al. [40] reported results from individual counselling of mastectomy patients. Two months after hospital discharge, the women were unchanged in mood but had greater internal locus of control that is usually associated with better adjustment.

Not many studies have evaluated individual therapy provided to late-stage cancer patients. Over a 3-year period, we [41] randomly assigned 120 men who were identified as having clinical stage IV cancer to individual therapy or usual medical treatment groups. Patients were seen several times a week. The objective was to develop a relationship of trust so that patients could talk freely. Efforts were made to reduce denial but maintain hope. Feelings of control over part of environment were stressed. Meaningful activities were encouraged for as long as possible. Listening to patients in what has been described as 'life review' helped to reinforce accomplishments, develop a sense of meaning to life, and provide the basis for increased self-esteem and life satisfaction. Simply listening, understanding, and sometimes only sitting quietly with patients were elements of therapy. Patients were assessed before random assignment and at 1, 3, 9, and 12 months, or for as long as the patient lived. Functional status and survival did not differ between groups; however, those who received therapy improved significantly over controls on depression, alienation, and life satisfaction within 3 months. Those living longer than 3 months maintained these same gains, except that levels of depression were similar between therapy and control groups after 3 months. By 9 months, those in therapy also showed more internal locus of control than did the controls. The results of the study were similar when a subgroup of 68 men with lung cancer (therapy and controls) were compared in the same way. In general, the study supported the hypothesis that quality of life was improved by individual counselling in terminally ill cancer patients.

In summary, results from studies of individual psychotherapy suggest that there is some benefit from treatment; however, findings vary. There is little evidence at this time that results from one type of intervention differ much from another type in helping patients with cancer, but that some supportive therapy generally reduces distress. The assumption that all cancer patients need therapy and that any type of therapy is better than no therapy is unjustified. Some patients may actually do worse in treatment than they would have without psychotherapeutic intervention. Further research is needed concerning which patients are at risk and which treatments are the most beneficial.

Selecting Patients for Therapy

It is estimated that one out of every three individuals in this country will experience cancer at some time. Not all of these patients need psychotherapy. Many of these individuals adjust in spite of prolonged treatments that disrupt their lives. In fact, a group of patients said to be cured of advanced cancers were found to have a zest for life and a sense of importance [42]. For some, cancer can be devastating. For others, a reasonably good adjustment is made to the disease. Worden and Weisman [43] suggested that three approaches or philosophies have been used in decisions about psychotherapeutic intervention. The first advocates providing treatment for everyone. The second suggests waiting to see who gets into serious emotional difficulties before treatment is offered. The third attempts to identify those at high risk so that preventive treatment can be provided before serious emotional problems develop. They have suggested that high-risk patients can be identified by mood, vulnerability as defined by factors such as alienation and denial, concerns about self and others, and problems in coping. A history of maladaptive coping with stressful events and a lack of social support in dealing with stressful events seem like relevant areas to explore as high-risk factors.

Models for Psychotherapeutic Interventions

Drawing on earlier studies of the role of loss and stressful life events as possible factors in cancer as well as the ongoing stress of cancer and its treatment, models for psychotherapy that are appropriate for stress reduction seem to be indicated. This is further confirmed by the finding that 68% of the DSM-III diagnoses found among cancer patients were those of adjustment disorders [17]. Criteria for diagnosing an adjustment disorder include: a maladaptive reaction to an identifiable stressor, with symptoms that occur within 3 months of the onset of the stressor and manifested by impaired social and occupational function; symptoms that are in excess of a normal reaction to stress, and reactions to stress that are not simply an exacerbation of some other mental disorder. It is also assumed that the disturbance will eventually remit after the stress ceases or, if the stressor persists, when a new level of adaptation is achieved. Whether a cancer patient meets criteria for a full-fledged diagnosis of an adjustment disorder or not, impaired coping with stress and reactions of depression may be signals that help is needed, particularly when there are few social supports to buffer against the effects of stress.

Crises intervention, as described by Caplan [44], Rapoport [45], and others, would appear to be one model for psychotherapy with cancer patients. It differs from other types of therapy in that it is time-limited, has well-defined goals that deal with relieving the immediate pain of the person in crises, and helps the person resume normal social functioning. The focus of therapy is always the resolution of the present crises. To aid the individuals in helping themselves, the therapist undertakes an assessment of the patients' social support systems and may even help to build social networks. Maladaptive goals are pointed out. Crises intervention is applicable when there is evidence of a precipitating event (in this case, cancer) that is related to the patient's present state of disequilibrium and when there is increased anxiety, emotional pain, and a breakdown of problem-solving skills. There should also be evidence that the patient is motivated to change in regard to coping behaviors.

Another model for therapy that might be applicable to cancer patients is that of brief dynamic psychotherapy as described by Horowitz et al. [46]. Stress response disorders occur in the context of life changes. Discrepancies between what is, what used to be, and what is wished for lead to emotional reactions. Anger, fear, sadness, and guilt may result. Brief dynamic psychotherapy uses the establishment of a therapeutic alliance to bolster the patient's sense of self-competence. As mastery is achieved, some of the negative symptoms tend to subside. This model of treatment has been successful with bereaved patients, a group with some of the same characteristics as those of cancer patients. Brief dynamic psychotherapy related the meaning intrinsic to changes in life circumstances to the individual's existing and current repertoire of self, his agendas for life, and his purposes and values. In treatment, the therapist regards the current symptoms as part of a life change toward a developmentally enhanced future. This optimistic stance treats any disorder, with its pain and suffering, as an opportunity for growth.

Because stress affects the characteristics of family relationships, family therapy, as described by Bowen [47] or Kerr [48], might be a treatment method of choice. Acute stress can produce changes in family relationships. Therapy requires working with the family as a unit. Family dysfunction or symptoms are identified. The focus is on helping each individual change rather than on encouraging family members to try to change one another. The emphasis is on emotional attachments as it is reflected in emotional distance and conflicts between family members. The therapist may see the family together or members individually. Because cancer disrupts interpersonal relationships in families, family therapy may be appropriate to help clarify and resolve the feelings of the family members.

A number of physical disorders, such as cancer, can produce maladaptive responses in emotionally healthy persons. Many times the physical impairment cannot be altered. Under such conditions, group therapy, as described by Lonergan [49], may help to facilitate adjustment by diminishing maladaptive coping patterns. There are several advantages of group therapy. Members can see themselves as having legitimate reactions to a stressor. Because all group members have the same problem (cancer), the focus for intervention is established quickly. The patients see they are not alone and can develop a sense of belonging and acceptance. Members can try out new behaviors for dealing with their problems in the group. Therapeutic elements of group therapy include interaction, cooperation, education, support, reinforcement, feedback, testing of perceptions, and modeling of behaviors as well as other elements specific to the individuals and their type of cancer. Cancer can be approached as an opportunity to reevaluate what is important in life and to take charge actively of those aspects of living that are most important. Groups may be used for short-term or long-term support. Long-term groups have been employed with terminally ill patients as well [50].

Stress management by behavioral methods, such as relaxation, somatic therapies, and cognitive behavioral therapies, offer promising models for treatment of cancer patients but are not reviewed here under the more traditional psychotherapeutic approaches.

Future Directions

Studies are needed that describe the rationale for selection of a particular model of treatment for well-defined groups of cancer patients, that describe elements of the treatment fully, and evaluate its effectiveness compared with control patients. Further analyses of responders versus nonresponders to treatment should help to define the characteristics of cancer patients that are the best candidates for a particular type of psychotherapy.

References

1 Bahnson, C.B.; Bahnson, M.B.: Role of the ego defenses: denial and repression in the etiology of malignant neoplasm. Ann. N.Y. Acad. Sci. *125:* 827–845 (1966).
2 Schmale, A.H.; Iker, H.P.: The affect of hopelessness in the development of cancer. I. The prediction of uterine cervical cancer in women with atypical cytology. Psychosom. Med. *26:* 634–635 (1964).
3 Kissen, D.: The significance of personality in lung cancer in men. Ann. N.Y. Acad. Sci. *125:* 820–826 (1966).

4 LeShan, L.: Psychological states as factors in the development of malignant disease: a critical review. J. natn. Cancer Inst. *22:* 1–18 (1959).
5 Temoshok, L. Fox, B.H.: Coping styles and other psychosocial factors related to medical status and to prognosis in patients with cutaneous malignant melanoma; in Fox, Newberry, Impact of psychoendocrine systems in cancer and immunity, pp. 258–287 (Hogrefe, Lewiston 1984).
6 Renneker, R.E.; Cutler, R.; Hora, J.; et al.: Psychoanalytical explorations of emotional correlates of cancer of the breast. Psychosom. Med. *25:* 106–123 (1963).
7 Goldberg, E.L.; Comstock, G.W.:Life events and subsequent illness. Am. J. Epidem. *104:* 146–158 (1976).
8 Lehrer, S.: Life change and gastric cancer. Psychosom. Med. *42:* 499–502 (1980).
9 Bartrop, R.; Luckhurst, E.; Lazarus, L.; Kiloh, L.; Penny, R.: Depressed lymphocyte function after bereavement. Lancet *i:* 834–836 (1977).
10 Locke, S.E.; Kraus, L.J.; Leserman, J.M.; Hurst, M.W.; Heisel, J.S.; Williams, R.M.: Life change stress, psychiatric symptoms, and natural killer cell activity. Psychosom. Med. *46:* 441–453 (1984).
11 Arnetz, B.B.; Wasserman, J.; Petrini, B.; Brenner, S.O.; Levi, L.; Eneroth, P.; Salovaara, H.; Hjelm, R.; Salovaara, L.; Theorell, T.; Petterson, I.L.: Immune function in unemployed women. Psychosom. Med.: *49:* 3–12 (1987).
12 Kiecolt-Glaser, J.K.; Fisher, L.D.; Ogrocki, P.; Stout, J.C.; Speicher, C.E.; Glaser, R.: Marital quality, marital disruption, and immune function. Psychosom. Med. *49:* 13–34 (1987).
13 Riley, V.; Spackman, D.H.; Hellstrom, K.E.; Hellstrom, I.: Growth enhancement of murine sarcoma by LDH-virus, adrenocorticoids, and anxiety stress. Proc. Am. Ass. Cancer Res. *19:* 57 (1978).
14 Riley, V.: Psychoneuroendocrine influences on immunocompetence and neoplasia. Science *212:* 1100–1109 (1981).
15 Scheifer, S.J.; Keller, S.E.; Meyerson, A.T.; Raskin, M.J.; Davis, K.L.; Stein, M.: Lymphocyte function in major depressive disorder. Archs gen. Psychiat. *41:* 484–486 (1984).
16 Whitlock, F.A.; Siskind, M.: Depression and cancer: a follow-up study. Psychol. Med. *9:* 747–752 (1979).
17 Derogatis, L.R.; Morrow, G.R.; Fetting, J.; Penman, D.; Piasetsky, S.; Schmale, A.M.; Henrichs, M.; Carnicke, C.L.M.: The prevalence of psychiatric disorders among cancer patients. J. Am. med. Ass. *249:* 751–757 (1983).
18 Plumb, M.M.; Holland, J.: Comparative studies of psychological functions in patients with advanced cancer. 1. Self-reported depressive symptoms. Psychosom. Med. *39:* 264–276 (1977).
19 Peck, A.: Emotional reactions to having cancer. Am. J. Roentg. *114:* 591–599 (1972).
20 Bukberg, J.; Penman, D.; Holland, J.C.: Depression in hospitalized cancer patients. Psychosom. Med. *46:* 199–212 (1984).
21 Stavraky, K.M.; Buck, C.N.; Lott, J.S.; Worklin, J.M.: Psychological factors in the outcome of human cancer. J. psychosom. Res. *12:* 251–259 (1968).
22 Blumberg, E.M.; West, P.M.; Ellis, F.W.: A possible relationship between psychological factors and human cancer. Psychosom. Med. *4:* 277–286 (1954).
23 Derogatis, L.R.; Abeloff, M.D.; Melisaratos, N.: Psychological coping mechanisms and survival time in metastatic breast cancer. J. Am. med. Ass. *242:* 1504–1508 (1979).

24 Greer, S.; Morris, T.; Pettingale, K.W.: Psychological response breast cancer: effect on outcome. Lancet *ii:* 785–787 (1979).
25 Watson, M.: Psychosocial intervention with cancer patients: a review. Psychol. Med. *13:* 839–846 (1983).
26 Bloom, J.R.; Ross, R.D.: Comprehensive psychosocial support for initial breast cancer: a preliminary report. Proc. Annu. Meet. Psychological Association, San Francisco 1977.
27 Spiegel, D.; Bloom, J.; Yalom, I.: Group support for patients with metastatic cancer. Archs gen. Psychiat. *38:* 527–533 (1981).
28 Weisman, A.D.; Worden, J.W.; Sobel, H.J.: Psychosocial screening and intervention with cancer patients. Unpubl. rep. Project Omega (Department of Psychiatry, Harvard Medical School, Cambridge 1980).
29 Blake, S.M.: Group psychotherapy with breast cancer patients: a controlled trial. Unpubl. M Sc thesis (Department of Psychiatry, University of Manchester, Manchester 1983).
30 Jacobs, C.; Ross, R.D.; Walker, I.M.; Stockdale, F.E.: Behavior of cancer patients: a randomized study of the effects of education and peer support groups. Am. J. clin. Oncol. *6:* 347–353 (1983).
31 Heinrich, R.L.; Schag, C.C.: Stress and activity management: group treatment for cancer patients and spouses. J. consult. clin. Psychol. *53:* 439–446 (1985).
32 Ferlic, M.; Goldman, A.; Kennedy, B.J.: Group counselling in adult patients with advanced cancer. Cancer *43:* 760–766 (1979).
33 Billings, A.G.; Moos, R.H.: Social support and functioning among community and clinical groups: a panel model. J. behav. Med. *5:* 295–312 (1982).
34 Kaplan, B.H.; Robbins, C.; Martin, S.S.: Antecedents of psychological stress in young adults: self-rejection, deprivation of social support, and life events. J. Health soc. Behav. *24:* 230–244 (1983).
35 Capone, M.A.; Good, R.S.; Westie, S.; Jacobson, A.F.:Psychosocial rehabilitation of gynaecological oncology patients. Archs Phys. med. Rehabil. *61:* 128 132 (1980).
36 Farash, J.L.: Effect of counselling on resolution of loss and body image disturbance following a mastectomy. Diss. Abstr. int. *38:* 4027 (1979).
37 Gordon, W.A.; Freidenbergs, I.; Diller, L.; Hibbard, M.; Wolf, C.; Levine, L.; Lipkins, R.; Ezrachi, O.; Lucido, D.: Efficacy of psychosocial intervention with cancer patients. J. consult. clin. Psychol. *48:* 743–759 (1980).
38 Watson, M.: Results of supportive therapy; in Stoll, Coping with cancer stress, pp. 123–129 (Nijhoff, Dordrecht 1986).
39 Forester, B.; Kornfeld, D.S.; Fleiss, J.L.: Psychotherapy during radiotherapy: effects on emotional and physical distress. Am. J. Psychiat. *142:* 22–27 (1985).
40 Bloom, J.R.; Ross, R.D.; Burnell, G.: The effect of social support on patient adjustment after breast surgery. Patient Counsell. Healt Educ. *Autumn:* 50–59 (1978).
41 Linn, M.V.; Linn, B.S.; Harris, R.: Effects of counseling for late stage cancer patients. Cancer *49:* 1048–1055 (1982).
42 Kennedy, B.J.; Tellegen, A.; Kennnedy, S. Havernick, N.: Psychological response of patients cured of advanced cancer. Cancer *38:* 2184–2191 (1976).
43 Worden, J.W.; Weisman, A.D.: Preventive psychosocial intervention with newly diagnosed cancer patients. Gen. Hosp. Psychiat. *6:* 243–249 (1984).
44 Caplan, G.: Principles of preventive psychiatry (Basic Books, New York 1964).

45 Rapoport, L.: The state of crises: some theoretical considerations. Soc. Serv. Rev. *36:* 211–217 (1962).
46 Horowitz, M.J.; Marmar, C.; Krupnick, J.; Wilner, N.; Kaltreider, N.; Wallerstein, R.: Personality styles and brief psychotherapy (Basic Books, New York 1984).
47 Bowen, M.: Family therapy in clinical practice (Aronson, New York 1978).
48 Kerr, M.: Emotional factors in the onset and course of cancer; in Sagar, Georgetown Family Symp. Washington 1979.
49 Lonergan, E.C.: Group intervention: how to begin and maintain groups in medical and psychiatric settings (Aronson, New York 1982).
50 Yalom, I.D.; Greaves, C.: Group therapy with the terminally ill. Am. J. Psychiat. *234:* 396–400 (1977).

Margaret W. Linn, PhD, Social Science Research, VA Medical Center,
1201 NW 16th Street, Miami, FL 33125 (USA)

Adv. psychosom. Med., vol. 18, pp. 66–81 (Karger, Basel 1988)

The Application of Behavior Therapy in Oncology

Anthony Spirito[a], *Kathy Hewett*[b], *Lori J. Stark*[b]

[a]Rhode Island Hospital, Brown University Program in Medicine, Providence, R.I.;
[b]Dana Farber Cancer Institute, Harvard Medical School, Boston, Mass., USA

The purpose of this chapter is to provide an overview of behavioral assessment and treatment strategies for pediatric and adult oncology patients. After outlining some of the basic principles of learning which underlie behavioral techniques, the remainder of the chapter will focus on specific problem areas associated, either directly or indirectly, with cancer and/or the treatment of cancer which have proved amenable to behavioral interventions.

Learning Theory and Symptom Formation

Classical Conditioning

Learning to respond to a neutral stimulus because it has been associated with another stimulus that elicits a response is the essential mechanism of classical conditioning. Classical conditioning has been suggested to play an important role in medical disorders which have symptoms that occur abruptly, in specific situations, create anxiety, and are not particularly affected by the environment [42]. For example, anticipatory nausea and vomiting may be especially susceptible to this type of learning. Chemotherapy drugs (the unconditioned stimulus) produce an aversive physiologic reaction, nausea and vomiting (unconditioned response). Over time, stimuli associated with chemotherapy, such as the treatment room or a particular nurse or doctor (conditioned stimulus), will result in the same aversive physiologic reaction, nausea and vomiting (conditioned response), as chemotherapy itself.

Operant Conditioning

In operant conditioning theory, a person will increase the performance of behaviors which are followed by positive or rewarding consequences and decrease those which are followed by aversive or punishing consequences. In medical disorders, some symptomatic behaviors may be influenced by operant conditioning factors. A prime example would be pain behavior. Increased attention to the patient from a parent or spouse and/or alleviation of chores, duties, etc. in response to pain complaints may lead to maladaptive coping styles such as avoidance. Another example has been presented by Reed [30] in which increased attention from family members and medical staff were found to be maintaining maladaptive behaviors of excessive crying and expressions of distress in a terminal cancer patient.

Since a variety of environmental stimuli may contribute to the development and maintenance of maladaptive behavior in the oncology patient, the ideas of Moxley [26] have been employed in an attempt to identify environmental factors of primary importance in hospital settings [32]. Three classes of factors are discussed: enduring setting events, temporary ongoing activity events, and pinpoint interaction events. Enduring setting events refer to naturally occurring stimuli, such as the nurses' call button, that lead to symptomatic behavior because of social reinforcement. These enduring setting events are problematic since they can encourage passivity and dependence on others. Temporary ongoing activity events, the second category, are much less predictable and include such things as a visit by attending staff or laboratory procedures which occur sporadically. Pinpointed interaction events refer to regularly occurring behavior, such as rounds by the attending physician or change of shifts in nursing staff. These events are important and need to be systematically assessed because they help to shape functional relationships between antecedent and consequent events, as well as desirable and undesirable behaviors in the hospital.

Although useful in understanding symptom presentation in oncology patients, a number of factors may interfere with interventions based on operant theory [32]. First, it is often difficult to determine whether a symptom has a physical or psychological basis since identical behaviors may be emitted in both cases. Second, hospital staff may find it difficult to confront a seriously ill patient with the impression that certain behaviors are related to secondary gain. They may have also had the experience of seeing patients with 'psychological' symptoms which were later found to have a bona fide organic basis and thus be reluctant to confront patients. Indeed, given the changing nature of symptoms in this population, ignoring pain behavior may be unwarranted and not constitute good medical care. Third, it is often difficult to ask hospital personnel to interact differently with patients since the demands of their job often take precedence over individually tailored treatment programs. And fourth, due to the numerous nursing personnel involved with patients, consistency among hospital personnel in implementing behavioral programs is often difficult to achieve.

Social Learning Theory

Social learning theory also accounts for numerous behavior patterns through observational learning (modeling) and self-regulatory processes. Modeling is a basic form of learning in which a behavior is acquired through the observation of another person engaging in that behavior. It is felt to be particularly important in the acquisition of various social behaviors. Modeling of pain behavior by family members and other patients may be particularly relevant in work with cancer patients.

Self-regulation depends upon an individual's ability to understand and modify antecedents, behavior, or the consequences of a particular behavior. Given the nature of cancer and its treatment, the oncology patient's ability to self-regulate can be substantially compromised as a result of both physiologic and psychologic stressors. Strengthening of previously utilized self-regulatory processes or teaching a patient new self-control processes can help overcome behavioral factors which may maintain maladaptive response patterns. If these self-control techniques are successful, they can lead to a primary change in a patient's feelings of self-efficacy.

While it is helpful to distinguish between classical conditioning, operant conditioning, and social learning theories, the clinician is often confronted with complex human behavior which requires both operant and classical conditioning as well as social learning to explain symptom patterns. Consequently, a thorough behavioral assessment should include all types of stimulus events including environmental stimuli, and the patient's own behavior, physiologic responses, and cognitions. Further, a variety of interventions should be employed as necessary to reduce the symptomatic behavior. In the sections that follow, some common problem areas encountered by behavioral clinicians working with cancer patients are discussed. Some of the major research studies in particular areas are reviewed but the sections are not intended to be a comprehensive overview of research. Instead, clinical details of selected treatment studies are discussed in depth in order to familiarize the reader with the nature of behavior therapy.

Problem Areas and Intervention

Pain

Pain is a significant problem encountered by health professionals working with oncology patients. The nature and extent of the problem is reflected in the number of surgical, medical, and pharmalogical interventions proposed for the treatment of cancer pain. Psychological factors have also begun to play a more important role in the health professions' thinking about all types of pain including cancer pain. In the past, a variety of psychological interventions, most centering around supportive psychotherapy for the anxiety and depression which may exacerbate perception of pain, have been employed. These psychological interventions were instituted, at least in part, for cancer patients who failed to benefit from the variety of medical treatments provided for pain relief. Studies have also underscored the significance of psychological factors of pain. In one study [3], placebos provided pain relief for 4 hours or more in approximately 77% of patients with advanced cancer. Given the importance of psychological factors in cancer pain, it is not surprising that a number of behavioral interventions have been proposed to help alleviate such pain.

Acute Pain

For assessment purposes, behavioral clinicians often conceptualize pain along at least two dimensions: chronic versus acute pain and disease-related versus treatment-related pain. In oncology patients acute pain responses are typically associated with the treatment while chronic pain responses are associated with the state of the disease. Of course, acute pain can be the result of disease. However, since disease-related acute pain is unpredictable in most patients, behavioral research and treatment has focused on interventions for acute pain states secondary to aversive medical procedures. While there are many oncology treatments which evoke acute pain, the present discussion will focus on pain associated with invasive procedures commonly used in treatment such as bone marrow aspirations and lumbar punctions. The pain resulting from such procedures is not primarily due to psychological factors, but certain behaviors and anxiety can play an important role in the distress experienced by cancer patients undergoing such treatment. Most of the clinical and controlled research studies on acute treatment-related pain have been conducted with children.

Hypnosis. Hypnosis to assist pediatric oncology patients in their coping with aversive medical procedures has been the most widely employed intervention to date. Some early uncontrolled clinical case studies [13] as well as a study reporting on the use of hypnosis and self-hypnosis for 27 childhood cancer patients [22] were the original reports to appear in the literature regarding the potential efficacy of hypnosis with pediatric oncology patients. Hilgard and LeBaron [15] were the first investigators to use a pre-post design in evaluating the effects of hypnosis on 24 children receiving bone marrow aspirations as part of their treatment for cancer. These authors reported that hypnosis was effective in helping increase the children's tolerance of these procedures. However, they did not include a control group in their design.

Another group of investigators [20] reported similar results with a sample of 16 adolescent cancer patients who were taught hypnotic procedures to help deal with the pain and distress that accompanied bone marrow aspirations or lumbar punctures and placement of IVs. The hypnotic procedure used by these investigators exemplifies that typically utilized by clinicians preparing patients for aversive medical procedures. These investigators began their hypnotic procedure by a short hypnotic induction such as an eye ball roll, eye fixation, or hand levitation technique. This induction was followed by a combination of systematic muscle tensing and relaxing and meditative breathing to help deepen the state of relaxation. Finally, when patients were judged to have achieved a reasonably good level of relaxation, they were instructed to imagine a favorite, calming place. The imagery techniques are believed to enhance the feeling of relaxation and deepen the hypnotic state. These authors also used a post-hypnotic suggestion at the end of their procedure. The post-hypnotic suggestion was for increased periods of comfort and well-being and diminished distress in the future during procedures. Although positive findings were found in the patient's self-report of anxiety and discomfort, objective behavioral observations were not conducted in this study.

Only one controlled outcome study has examined the efficacy of hypnosis for pain in childhood cancer patients [43]. In this study 33 cancer patients between the ages of 6 and 17 were assigned to either hypnosis training or nonhypnotic behavioral training for use with aversive medical procedures (bone marrow aspirations and spinal taps). Both patient self-report and behavior ratings by independent observers were used to evaluate outcome of the training. In the hypnosis group, patients were trained in the use of individually tailored imagery and fantasy combined with some meditative breathing. In the nonhypnotic group, a combination of deep breathing, distraction, and practice sessions to help control anxiety were used. Imagery focusing on distraction rather than fantasy was also employed. The hypnotic intervention was found to be more effective than the non-hypnotic intervention for both bone marrows and lumbar punctures. The authors speculate that the hypnosis condition was more powerful due to the fact that the images employed were better able to hold the child's attention.

From the studies reviewed above, it is reasonable to conclude that hypnosis may be an effective intervention for acute pain arising secondary to aversive medical procedures. However, not all patients respond equally well to hypnotic intervention. This is a function of both patient and therapist characteristics. There have been a number of articles and books written about hypnotherapy with children which address the clinical characteristics which dictate success with such intervention [8, 14–16]. The reader is referred to these sources in order to get a better understanding of relevant characteristics. Finally, although the literature with acute pain experience is almost exclusively with children, there is no reason to expect that similar procedures would not be effective with adult oncology patients since hypnosis has been employed for a number of other acute pain conditions with adults.

Cognitive Behavioral Techniques. In addition to hypnosis, a number of investigators have examined the efficacy of nonhypnotic cognitive behavioral packages for children coping with procedure-related pain. Jay et al. [17–19] have done the most work in this area and their approach exemplifies such an intervention. These investigators use a multicomponent intervention package specifically for children undergoing bone marrow aspirations and lumbar punctures. In order to reduce children's distress, five components are employed: filmed modeling, breathing training, imagery/distraction, behavioral rehearsal, and positive reinforcement. Their initial study with 5 childhood cancer patients indicated that such a package significantly reduced behavioral distress. Consequently, in a three-year controlled outcome study [cited in ref. 17] with 55 cancer patients between the ages of 4 and 14, this package has been employed to significantly reduce not only behavioral distress but the self-report of pain and physiologic arousal during bone marrow aspirations. The package was compared to a Valium sedation condition and a minimal treatment attention control group. The findings indicated that the cognitive behavioral intervention was significantly more effective than the other treatment groups. It was found that the Valium helped reduce distress prior to the procedure but was not as effective as the cognitive-behavioral technique during the procedure itself.

Whether hypnosis or cognitive behavioral training is employed, it seems that they can be reasonably effective approaches to dealing with the acute pain experienced by oncology patients. In fact, there is often much overlap between interventions labeled as hypnosis and those labeled as cognitive/behavioral. This overlap includes the use of some form of relaxation, the use of imagery, motivation enhancement by the therapist, and social reinforcement by the therapist. Whether hypnosis or a cognitive behavioral technique is used, motivation is a prime requirement for the techniques to be effective. Since self-hypnotic procedures are, by definition, taught to patients, the ultimate efficacy of the intervention lies in the hands of the patients themselves.

Chronic Pain

Chronic pain in cancer patients most often occurs secondary to progressive disease states. Such pain is often only mildly responsive to a variety of medical and surgical interventions. In addition, there often arises a number of secondary changes in behavior which impair the patient's daily functioning and lower the patient's ability to tolerate disease-related pain. These associated behaviors can include sleep and appetite disturbance, decreased activity, depression and anxiety, heightened attention to bodily sensations which increase the patient's perception of pain [28], and increased attention from family and medical staff secondary to pain complaints.

Two types of intervention for chronic pain which develops secondary to disease are usually employed: pain perception regulation and pain behavior regulation. Pain perception regulation is employed to provide self-control skills, e.g. relaxation and to help the cancer patient attenuate some of the pain experienced. Pain behavior regulation, which focuses on those environmental events which contribute to the expression of pain behavior and decrease opportunity for facilitating adaptive functioning, is also a focus of intervention where appropriate. The self-regulatory and operant interventions described previously for acute pain can be used for both acute and chronic pain conditions as well as treatment-related and disease-related pain. Thus, the reader should not be misled by the fact that greater discussion of self-regulatory processes is included under the acute pain section. More detailed reviews of the variety of behavioral interventions available for pain [36, 38, 39] and specifically of the research on behavioral interventions for pain in oncology patients can be found elsewhere [17].

The published literature on behavioral interventions for the chronic pain of cancer is almost entirely limited to adults. Research with adult patients consists of case histories and clinical reports rather than more rigorous methodological studies with control groups and objective assessment measures. Thus, the material that follows on the chronic pain of cancer is rather limited.

Hypnosis. Apparently only one controlled outcome study of hypnosis for disease-relate pain in cancer patients has been conducted [34]. In this study, women with metastatic breast cancer were assigned to a control group or to one of two weekly support groups. One of the support groups utilized self-hypnosis as an intervention for pain. Self-hypnosis training was brief and limited to the last 5–10 min of the group sessions. The hypnotic procedure involved having patients imagine a competing sensation with the pain, usually numbness, warmth, or a tingling sensation. The efficacy of these interventions was assessed using self-report methodology. The results of the study indicated that both intervention groups had smaller increases in pain over time than the control group. The hypnosis group had the lowest mean rating of pain increase but it is unclear whether their performance was significantly better than the other treatment group.

Cognitive-Behavioral Interventions. Cognitive-behavioral interventions for chronic pain would appear to hold much promise for the cancer patient. In these interventions, a variety of skills are taught to the patients to help them manage pain. The interventions can include cognitive restructuring, specific coping skills training, and the use of self-regulation techniques, such as relaxation training. The use of a multicomponent package in the case of chronic cancer pain is intuitively quite attractive. If one examines the different interventions employed in such a program, it seems clear that these complementary interventions may have an additive effect and may affect different symptoms simultaneously. For example, relaxation training employed may reduce emotional arousal and thereby aid in the patient's pain perception. At the same time, relaxation may have an effect on physiological arousal, i.e. muscle tension, that might be misinterpreted as cancer-related pain or might contribute to pain through muscle contraction.

Biofeedback is often employed in multicomponent training programs to enhance relaxation. Biofeedback entails the use of sensitive electronic equipment to monitor and amplify physiologic activity, such as muscle activity or peripheral temperature, in the form of a visual or auditory signal. These signals are then used to provide feedback to the patient about his/her own physiology. For more detailed discussion of clinical issues in biofeedback, see Shellenberger and Green [33].

One study [11] has looked at the effectiveness of both electromyographic (EMG) and electroencephalographic (EEG) feedback for reducing chronic pain in 7 cancer patients. In this series of case studies, a number of psychological and physiological variables were employed as dependent measures. Within-session changes on several dependent measures were noted reliably by the patients. Unfortunately, generalization outside the training sessions was not particularly evident for the patients.

Although, to our knowledge, no data has been published on a cognitive behavioral multicomponent program with chronic cancer pain, Turk and Rennert [37] describe such a program. Interested readers should refer to this detailed description to get a better understanding of the nature of such an intervention.

Treatment-Related Distress: Nausea, Vomiting, and Anxiety

Among the side effects which may occur as a result of cancer treatment, many patients have identified the nausea and vomiting associated with chemotherapy as the most distressing. Generally, nausea and vomiting during and following chemotherapy are a direct result of these drugs. Over the course of treatment, however, changes occur in immune system response, overall health status, expectations and experience with chemotherapy, and in the emotional responses associated with cancer treatment and the illness itself. Through the interaction of these factors, patients may develop conditioned responses to chemotherapy which include protracted or severe nausea and vomiting following chemotherapy. In addition, a significant subset of patients who experience post-chemotherapy sickness develop symptoms of discomfort, nausea, vomiting, and anxiety prior to administration of chemotherapy drugs. Recent prospective studies with adults and children have yielded consistent estimates that approximately 25–33% of adult and pediatric patients experience moderate to severe nausea prior to chemotherapy. Some 11–20% experience vomiting prior to chemotherapy. Evidence of anticipatory anxiety is consistently higher for all patients, with estimates around 60% for pediatric and adult patients.

Considerable attention has been paid to the role of personality and emotional factors in the development of conditioned responses to chemotherapy. The classical conditioning model developed for anticipatory nausea and vomiting (ANV) allows the potential for cognitive mediation of the conditioning process. That is, it is possible that individual differences in cognitive style (e.g. introverted personality style), or emotional states (e.g. heightened anxiety) contribute to the conditioning or learned responsivity. Since a noncognitive model cannot fully account for the variation among individuals in the rate and severity of symptom development or in the utility of antiemetic drugs, a mediating role for emotional states or personality style has acquired increased credibility in explaining the conditioned responses, especially of ANV.

The rationale and goals for using specific behavioral techniques in treating nausea and vomiting following directly from the classical conditioning model of symptom development. Behavioral techniques may be designed to: (1) Reduce autonomic arousal and thereby producing a physical state incompatible with the characteristic of nausea and vomiting. Reduction in autonomic arousal may also reduce autonomic cues available for conditioning. (2) Change or reduce pairings of chemotherapy with environmental stimuli. (3) Reduce post-chemotherapy nausea and vomiting, thus reducing a reliable predictor of anticipatory symptoms. (4) Change cognitions and perceptions concerning chemotherapy treatment, as well as self-control and coping strategies. (5) Reduce state anxiety (both cognitions and autonomic arousal features) typically associated with chemotherapy.

With the exception of using distraction with videogames to control nausea and vomiting among pediatric oncology patients [21], most studies with children and adults have employed either hypnosis or relaxation training as the primary behavioral techniques to address chemotherapy-related distress. Since these treatment modalities are employed in a manner similar to interventions with pain, interested readers should consult review articles [31] and some of the more well-known intervention studies [2, 7, 23, 25, 27, 44] for further details. The work of Burish [2, 6] will be reviewed as an example of the type of intervention employed.

Burish and colleagues [2, 6] have tested a behavioral intervention to reduce nausea/vomiting during and after chemotherapy. In this approach patients are taught muscle relaxation techniques and the use of a relaxing image in distracting themselves from the discomforts of treatment and in maintaining a low-arousal state. Training is begun prior to or just after the initial chemotherapy treatment with up to four subsequent training sessions by a therapist. Patients practice between courses of chemotherapy. When designing interventions for individual patients, behavioral clinicians can employ one of several relaxation techniques, i.e. imagery, progressive muscle relaxation, meditative breathing, etc. Experienced clinicians who employ relaxation techniques can also point to a number of factors, e.g. the use of words, timing, etc., which can significantly enhance the effects of the relaxation procedure. More detailed discussion of various relaxation procedures can be found in Fuller [12].

Studies with adults by Burish et al. [2] showed that patients were able to reduce the severity of nausea and vomiting during and after chemotherapy. They also were able to reduce their autonomic arousal as measured by pulse rate and blood pressure. Such reductions were not consistently maintained, however, when therapists were not present to help with the intervention. These authors also found that patients with high levels of baseline anxiety were less likely to benefit from behavioral training than those with moderate or low levels of baseline anxiety [6].

Sleep

Sleep difficulties which arise secondary to cancer treatment are a common complaint noted among clinicians working with oncology patients. In a survey of five major cancer treatment centers, it was found that 44% of all psychotropic drug prescriptions were written for sleep difficulties [9]. Although there have been many studies reported in the literature which have examined the effectiveness of behavioral techniques for a variety of sleep problems [40] only a few studies specifically focus on treatment with cancer patients. One study [5] reported on 15 adult cancer patients with sleep onset insomnia who were taught relaxation training. Daily training sessions were held over 3 consecutive days for each of these patients. When comparing the efficacy of this approach to a group of patients receiving routine care, relaxation training was found to significantly reduce sleep onset latency immediately following treatment and at a 3-month follow-up. Unfortunately, the treatment did not affect the number of hours slept by the intervention group.

More recently, a case study of a 27-year-old man who developed severe insomnia while being treated for cancer has been reported [35]. The man reported a 2-year history of sleep difficulties which were exacerbated by the death of a close friend and his own diagnosis of cancer. More specifically, the man noted that he was unable to sleep for more than a few hours in a row during the night. In addition, he never slept more than 6 h in the night and there were many nights when he slept no longer than 1 or 2 h. Prior treatment with medication had been stopped by the patient himself due to ineffectiveness.

Two of the more common behavioral techniques for insomnia were used in this study: somatic focusing and imagery training. During the somatic focusing training, the young man was asked to focus on feelings of tension in the 16 major muscle groups to release that tension without first tensing his muscles. He was asked to imagine his muscles becoming limp and heavy and then to imagine feelings of relaxation replacing tension. Following somatic focusing, the patient was asked to concentrate on specific features, color, and movement of common objects during imagery training. The patient was asked to visualize each object for several minutes while the trainer provided guided imagery instructions that were gradually faded out. In addition to the in-session training, the client was asked to practice at home daily. By session 5, this patient's duration of sleep had risen to about 7 h. A 12-month follow-up supported the long-term effectiveness of the intervention. This single case study suggests that clinicians familiar with behavioral interventions can effectively treat cancer patients who develop sleep difficulties. Indeed, it seems that sleep problems should be assessed more comprehensibly in cancer patients so that more effective interventions can be delivered for those patients experiencing sleep difficulties.

Anorexia

A number of different factors have been proposed to account for poor oral intake and weight gain among cancer patients. These include learned taste aversion secondary to chemotherapy, the disease itself interfering with the patient's ability to utilize nutrients, e.g. through changes in metabolism or obstructions, vomiting and diarrhea secondary to treatment, fatigue and nausea eliminating a patient's desire to eat, swallowing difficulties, pain, and anxiety and depression, secondary to the disease [4].

Eating difficulties among oncology patients have been found in both children and adults. One of the first studies [22] used hypnosis for children with cancer to aid in a variety of cancer-related side effects. One of the problems that was addressed was poor appetite and weight loss. In this uncontrolled study, the authors report that hypnosis was effective in increasing appetite and promoting weight gain. Operant techniques, such as behavioral reinforcement programs with rewards contingent on oral intake, are also commonly used with children and often quite effective.

In adults, two case studies have been reported in the literature and provide examples of typical behavioral approaches for eating difficulties. A case study [29] has been reported of a 53-year-old woman who presented with almost total inability to eat food over a 6-week period following an esophagogastrectomy for carcinoma of the stomach. Following the surgical procedure, the patient continued to report discomfort and anxiety about her disease while swallowing food which resulted in gagging and regurgitating almost continuously following eating. Intervention consisted of daily relaxation training followed by attempts to eat small amounts of selected foods. She gradually began to eat reasonably well and was discharged 19 days after the program had been implemented. A 9-month follow-up indicated the patient was still eating well. This simple program demonstrated that the anxiety-driven behaviors which interfere with eating could be quickly and easily limited so that the patient could begin to eat reasonably well.

Another single-case study of a 54-year-old man who completed a year-and-a-half of chemotherapy (cisplatinum and cytotoxin) following a prostectomy has also been published [41]. Upon referral, this man had lost 47 pounds (22.5% of his original body weight) over the previous year. He reported no desire for food and feelings of nausea upon sight, smell, or even mention of certain foods. The patient's diet was limited to liquids or soft foods usually served by his wife but eaten alone. The patient routinely vomited following eating and argued with family members who tried to get him to eat more. Fifteen behavioral treatment sessions were conducted over a 13-week period with this man. Treatment consisted of systematic desensitization, conducted over a 5-week period, using a hierarchical presentation of scenes in which the patient consumed liquids. After the patient had progressed to the point where an image did not produce sensations of nausea for three consecutive presentations, he was instructed to use imagery by himself and then to try to consume some of these fluids at home. By session 6, a cognitive restructuring procedure was also used in which some of the patient's negative self-statements were substituted with more adaptive coping statements. To complement this cognitive work, a contract was developed between the patient and his wife so that the patient could be more in control of his food intake and arguments about eating restricted. This intervention resulted in increased intake of a greater variety of foods although not an increase in caloric intake.

Campbell et al. [4] report on a study in which 22 persons with cancer were assigned to relaxation training to promote normal food consumption. Relaxation procedures included meditative breathing, deep muscle relaxation, and imagery. In this study, 75% of the patients who complied with relaxation training experienced a positive weight gain over a 6-week period while performance status as measured by the Karnofsky Scale improved for 33% of the group. Although the data was inconclusive since no control group was used, the study is significant for two reasons. First, some of the patients in the group reported that relaxation seemed to be related to their increased oral intake. In addition, of the 22 persons originally in the group, 10 did not comply with the home relaxation practice. This points out that in many of the self-control techniques used in behavioral interventions, whether they be for eating difficulties or other problems such as anxiety or pain, patient characteristics are important to assess prior to intervening. Motivation and expectation are important variables mediating the success of any of these treatments which require effort on the patients' part to lead to a favorable response.

Conclusions

Clinical and research findings on the utility of behavioral interventions in oncology are encouraging. However, a number of important clinical research questions remain unanswered and will prove important to investigate in the future. Although the methods of treatment have much in common across the different problem areas, therapy should always be tailored to the individual and based on a thorough assessment. As medical treatments improve in the future, problems arising secondary to treatment and the chronic nature of cancer will likely increase the role of behavioral interventions. Through the collaborative efforts of behavioral clinicans and oncologists, the potential for optimizing the overall care of cancer patients will be greatly increased.

References

1 Burish, T.; Carey, M.: Conditioned responses to cancer chemotherapy: etiology and treatment; in Fox, Newberry, Impact of psychoendocrine systems in cancer and immunity (Hogrefe, Toronto 1984).

2 Burish , T.; Carey, M.; Krozely, M.; Greco, F.: Conditioned side effects induced by cancer chemotherapy: prevention through behavioral treatment. J. consult. clin. Psychol. *55:* 42–48 (1987).

3 Byron, R.; Yonemoto, R.: Pain associated with malignancy; in Bonica, Ventafridda, Advances in pain research and therapy, vol. 2 (Raven Press, New York 1979).

4 Campbell, D.; Dixon, J.; Sanderford, L.; Penicola, M.: Relaxation: its effect on the nutritional status and performance status of clients with cancer. Am. diet. Ass. *84:* 201–204 (1984).

5 Cannici, J.; Malcolm, R.; Peek, L.: Treatment of insomnia in cancer patients using muscle relaxation training. J. Behav. Ther. exp. Psychiat. *14:* 251–256 (1983).

6 Carey, M.; Burish, T.: Anxiety as a predictor of behavioral therapy outcome for cancer chemotherapy patients. J. consult. clin. Psychol. *53:* 860–865 (1985).

7 Cotanch, P.; Hockenberry, M.; Herman, S.: Self-hypnosis as antiemetic therapy in children receiving chemotherapy. Onc. Nurs. For. *12:* 41–46 (1985).

8 Dash, J.: Hypnosis for symptom amelioration; in Kellerman, Psychological aspects of childhood cancer (Thomas, Springfield 1980).

9 Derogatis, L.; Feldstein, M.; Morrow, G.; Schmale, A.; Schmitt, M.; Gates, C.; Murawski, B.; Holland, J.; Penman, D.; Melisarotos, N.; Enelow, A.; McKinney, L.: A survey of psychotropic drug prescriptions in an oncology population. Cancer *44:* 1919–1929 (1979).
10 Dolgin, M.; Katz, E.; McGinty, K.; Siegel, S.: Anticipatory nausea and vomiting in pediatric cancer patients. Pediatrics *75:* 547–552 (1985).
11 Fotopoulos, S.; Graham, C.; Cook, M.: Psychophysiologic control of cancer pain; in Bonica, Ventafridda, Advances in pain research and therapy, vol. 2 (Raven Press, New York 1979).
12 Fuller, G.: Biofeedback: methods and procedures in clinical practice (Biofeedback Press, San Francisco 1977).
13 Gardner, G.: Childhood, death and human dignity: hypnotherapy for David. Int. J. clin. exp. Hypnosis *24:* 122–139 (1976).
14 Gardner, G.; Olness, K.: Hypnosis and hypnotherapy with children (Grune & Stratton, New York 1981).
15 Hilgard, E.; LeBaron, S.: Relief of anxiety and pain in children and adolescents with cancer: quantitative measures and clinical observations. Int. J. clin. exp. Hypnosis *30:* 417-442 (1982).
16 Hilgard, J.; LeBaron, S.: Hypnotherapy of pain in children with cancer (Kaufman, Los Altos 1984).
17 Jay, S.; Elliott, C.; Varni, J.: Acute and chronic pain in adults and children with cancer. J. consult. clin. Psychol. *54:* 601–607 (1986).
18 Jay, S.; Elliott, C.; Katz, E.; Siegel, S.: Cognitive-behavioral intervention for children undergoing painful medical procedures: final results of a treatment outcome study; in Varni, Comprehensive assessment and management of acute and chronic pain in children. Symposium conducted at the Annual Meeting of the Association for the Advancement of Behavior Therapy, Houston 1985.
19 Jay, S.; Elliot, C.; Ozolins, M.; Pruitt, S.: Behavioral management of childrens' distress during painful medical procedures. Behav. Res. Therapy *23:* 513–520 (1985).
20 Kellerman, J.; Zeltzer, L.; Ellenberg, L.; Dash, J.: Adolescents with cancer: hypnosis for the reduction of acute pain and anxiety associated with medical procedures. J. adolesc. Health Care *4:* 85–90 (1983).
21 Kolko, D.; Richard-Figueroa, J.: Effects of videogames on the adverse corollaries of chemotherapy in pediatric oncology patients: a single-case analysis. J. consult. clin. Psychol. *53:* 223–228 (1985).
22 LaBaw, W.; Holton, C.; Tewell, K.; Eccles, D.: The use of self-hypnosis by children with cancer. Am. J. clin. Hypnosis *17:* 233-238 (1975).
23 LeBaron, S.; Zeltzer, L.: Behavioral intervention for reducing chemotherapy-related nausea and vomiting in adolescents with cancer. J. adolesc. Health Care *5:* 178–182 (1984).
24 Morrow, G.: Prevalence and correlates of anticipatory nausea and vomiting induced by cancer chemotherapy. J. natn. Cancer Inst. *68:* 585–588 (1982).
25 Morrow, G.; Morrell, C.: The antiemetic efficacy of behavioral treatment for cancer chemotherapy induced anticipatory nausea and vomiting: standardized trial of systematic desensitization, counselling placebo, and no treatment. New Engl. J. Med. *307:* 1476–1480 (1982).
26 Moxley, R.: Graphics for three-term contingencies. Behav. Anal. *5:* 45–51 (1982).
27 Olness, K.: Imagery (self-hypnosis) as adjunct therapy in childhood cancer. Clinical experience with 25 patients. Am. J. Ped. Hematol. Oncol. *3:* 313–321 (1981).

28 Pilowsky, I.; Chapman, C.; Bonica, J.: Pain, depression, and illness behavior in a pain clinic population. Pain. *4:* 183–192 (1977).
29 Redd, W.H.: In vivo desensitization in the treatment of chronic emesis following gastrointestinal surgery. Behav Ther. *11:* 421–427 (1980).
30 Redd, W.: Treatment of excessive crying in a terminal cancer patient: a time-series analysis. Behav. Mod. *5:* 225–236 (1982).
31 Redd, W.; Andrykowski, M.: Behavioral intervention in cancer treatment: controlling aversion reactions to chemotherapy. J. consult. clin. Psychol. *50:* 1018–1029 (1982).
32 Redd, W.; Rusch, F.: Behavioral analysis in behavioral medicine. Behav. Mod. *9:* 131–154 (1985).
33 Shellenberg, R.; Green, J.: From the ghost in the box to successful biofeedback training. (Health Psychology Publication, Greeley 1986).
34 Spiegel, D.; Bloom, J.: Group therapy and hypnosis reduce metastatic breast carcinoma pain. Psychosom. Med. *45:* 333–339 (1983).
35 Stam, H.; Bultz, B.: The treatment of severe insomnia in a cancer patient. J. Behav. Ther. exp. Psychiat. *17:* 33–37 (1986).
36 Tan, S.: Cognitive and cognitive-behavioral methods for pain control: a selective review. Pain *12:* 201–228 (1982).
37 Turk, D.; Rennert, K.: Pain and the terminally ill cancer patient: a cognitive-social learning perspective; in Sobel, Behavior therapy in terminal care (Ballinger, Cambridge 1981).
38 Turner, J.; Chapman, C.: Psychological intervention for chronic pain: a critical review. I. Relaxation training and biofeedback. Pain *12:* 1–21 (1982).
39 Turner, J.; Chapman, C.: Psychological intervention for chronic pain: a critical review. II. Operant conditioning, hypnosis, and cognitive-behavioral therapy. Pain *12:* 23-46 (1982).
40 Turner, R.; DiTomasso, R.: The behavioral treatment of insomnia: a review and methodological analyses of the evidence. Int. J. ment. Health *9:* 129-148 (1980).
41 West, B.; Goethe, K.; Piccionne, C.: Cognitive-behavioral techniques in treating anorexia and depression in a cancer patient. Behav. Ther. *5:* 115–117 (1982).
42 Whitehead, W.; Fedoravicius, A.; Blackwell, B.; Wooley, S.: A behavioral conceptualization of psychosomatic illness: psychosomatic symptoms as learned responses; in MacNamara, Behavioral approaches to medicine: application and analysis (Plenum Press, New York 1979).
43 Zeltzer, L.; LeBaron, S.: Hypnosis and nonhypnotic techniques for reduction of pain and anxiety during painful procedures in children and adolescent with cancer. J. Pediat. *101:* 1032–1035 (1982).
44 Zeltzer, L.; LeBaron, S.; Zeltzer, P.: The effectiveness of behavioral intervention for reduction of nausea and vomiting in children and adolescents receiving chemotherapy. J. clin. Oncol. *2:* 683–690 (1984).

Anthony Spirito, PhD, Rhode Island Hospital, Brown University Program in Medicine, 593 Eddy Street, Providence, RI 02903 (USA)

Adv. psychosom. Med., vol. 18, pp. 82–101 (Karger, Basel 1988)

Family Issues in Cancer Care

Laurel L. Northouse

College of Nursing, Wayne State University, Detroit, Mich., USA

Cancer presents a crisis for patients but it also presents a crisis for family members. Cancer is often called a 'family disease' because of its immediate impact on family functioning, roles, and relationships [1]. Although cancer has a stressful effect on the whole family, most of the research in this area has focused only on patients. As a result, health professionals have a limited understanding of the impact of cancer on the entire family and of the interventions that could be used to assist family members to cope with the effects of illness.

The purpose of this chapter is to review the research that has been conducted with family members of adult cancer patients. The chapter has been divided into four sections: (1) cancer and family stress; (2) cancer and intrafamily relations; (3) cancer and family caregiving responsibilities, and (4) cancer and family-professional relationships. The chapter concludes with implications for clinical practice.

Cancer and Family Stress

Family systems theory provides a useful theoretical framework for understanding the impact of cancer on patients and family members. The concept of the family as a system emphasizes the interrelatedness among family members and the mutual effect that they have on one another [2, 3]. Changes that occur in one part of the family system are accompanied by compensatory changes in another part of the system. From a systems perspective, when illness occurs in the family, the effects are not confined to the sick individual but reverberate throughout the family.

The diagnosis of cancer can generate considerable anxiety and tension within the family. For many years family members were considered immune to the stress of the patients's illness. Since family members did not have physical symptoms of the disease, they were considered insulated and protected from its effects. In recent years, however, a small but growing body of research has emerged that has documented the stressful impact of the patient's cancer on family members. This section of the chapter will describe the nature of family members' stress, the magnitude of their stress, and factors related to their stress.

Nature of Family Members' Stress

One of the landmark studies on the impact of cancer on family members was conducted by Wellisch et al. [4] in 1978. These investigators found that husbands of breast cancer patients reported significant psychosomatic and psychological difficulties at the time of their wives' surgery and up to the time the patients were discharged from the hospital. Among the difficulties reported by husbands, most pronounced were problems with sleep, loss of appetite, and a decreased ability to concentrate at work.

Similar psychosomatic concerns have been reported by other family members, as well as problems with heightened anxiety and the exacerbation of various illnesses. Welch [5], for example, reported that 27% of the family members acknowledged the intensification of headaches, sleeping problems, eating problems, and other physical problems after the onset of their family members's cancer. Lovejoy [6] found that 75% of the family members reported anxiety and also problems with worry, fatigue, and insomnia. In addition, some family members reported the development of other physical problems such as hypertension and chest pains following the patient's diagnosis.

The stress experienced by family members occurs during all phases of the illness. In the diagnostic phase, family members often experience shock, uncertainty, and a tremendous release of emotions. This is often followed by exhaustion as they no longer have the strength or the resources to cope with the stress surrounding the diagnostic period [6, 7]. In the recurrent phase, family members report intense fear and anger because the cure they assumed the patient had is suddenly interrupted by the return of the disease [8]. Uncertainty is also prevalent during this time as family members worry about the effectiveness of cancer treatments and the patient's survival. In the terminal phase, family members report despair and isolation as they watch their loved one suffer [9]. Family members also report feelings of helplessness and loss as death approaches [10]. During each phase of cancer family members must grapple with the effects of the illness.

Magnitude and Duration of Stress

How much stress do family members report and how long does it last? There is some indication that the level of stress experienced by family members is comparable to the level of stress reported by patients. Northouse and Swain [11], for example, compared the mood and distress scores of 50 mastectomy patients and their husbands 3 days after surgery and again 30 days later and found no significant differences between patients' and husbands' mood and distress scores. Husbands reported as much distress as their wives during the hospitalization period and 30 days after the patient returned home. In addition, both patients and husbands had levels of distress that were above the mean for the normal population. Cassileth et al. [12], also comparing the anxiety and moodf states of cancer patients and relatives, found that their scores were not only similar but highly correlated. In the study by Baider and Kaplan De-Nour [13] patients' and spouses' adjustment scores were also correlated. Patients with high levels of distress had husbands with high levels of distress. Conversely, patients with lower levels of distress had husbands who experienced less distress.

The magnitude of the distress reported by family members apears closer to the profile of the normal poulation than that of the psychiatric population. Plumb and Holland [14] reported that cancer patients and their next of kin were indistinguishable in terms of their level of psychological depression, yet both had depression scores that were significantly lower than the scores of patients hospitalized for suicide attempts. Similarly, Northouse and Swain [11] found that mastectomy patients and their husbands reported more distress than the general population, but the average distress scores for patients and husbands were well below the mean scores for psychiatric patients. The clinical relevance of these comparisons suggests that strategies to assist family members with stress need to be geared more toward a general population that is stressed by the cancer experience rather than toward a psychiatric population with intrapsychic problems.

Although documentation is limited concerning how long family members experience the stressful effects of cancer, a few longitudinal studies indicate that the effects on family members are not transient but continue for an extended period of time. Maguire [15] compared the distress levels of 52 husbands of mastectomy patients with husbands of women with benign breast disease at three points in time: prior to surgery, 3 months after surgery, and one year after surgery. Husbands of mastectomy patients reported significantly more distress than the control group at each of the assessment times. At one year post surgery, husbands of mastectomy patients reported significantly more anxiety, more sexual difficulties, and more problems at work (e.g. decreased concentration) than husbands of women with benign breast disease. Oberst and James [7] found that family members' stress waxes and wanes over the course of illness. They found that spouses' anxiety and distress levels were high just prior to the patients' discharge from the hospital, lower after the patient returned home (when the spouse was on familiar turf), and then rose again 60 days later.

Factors Related to Family Members' Stress

Given that family members experience significant amounts of stress, what are some of the factors that may contribute to their stress? One factor appears to be the pervasive sense of helplessness that arises when a loved one is diagnosed with cancer. Watching the patient suffer and not knowing how to alleviate the suffering has been reported as a major problem by family members [10, 16, 17]. Spouses of lung cancer patients, for example, reported feeling helpless as 'they stood empty-handed and watched their mates deteriorate' [18]. Vachon et al. [9] compared the stress and adjustment problems of widows of cancer patients and widows of cardiac patients. Widows of cancer patients reported more stress, more helplessness, and more feelings of impotence than widows of cardiac patients. Whereas widows of cardiac patients felt they could help their husbands by attending to their diets and activity needs, widows of cancer patients felt there was little that they could do to alter the course of the disease.

Another factor that contributes to family members' stress is the fear that accompanies the diagnosis of cancer. Even though many advances have been made in the treatment of cancer, many people still equate cancer with death. Gotay [19] found that the most common concern reported by both cancer patients and their mates was their fear of the disease. Fear was ranked as the number one response of family members of patients in both early and advanced stages of cancer. Family members reported specific fears about the potential progression and recurrence of the disease.

There is some indication that treatment characteristics are also related to family members' levels of distress. Cassileth et al. [12, p. 75] found that family members of patients receiving active treatment reported significantly more anxiety and mood disturbances than family members of patients receiving follow-up care. Furthermore, family members of patients receiving palliative care reported the highest levels of distress. According to the investigators, relatives of patients receiving cancer treatment have not yet attained a sense of security and 'are faced also with fears, inconvenience, treatment-related toxicity, and massive uncertainty'.

A fourth factor related to stress of family members is the lack of supportive resources. Spouses, in a study by Oberst and James [7], reported anger and frustration about the lack of support they perceived from all sources including professionals. One spouse said:

> Nobody understands what I'm going through. He's feeling better and I keep feeling worse. Everyone pats him on the back and says how well he's managing. No one asks about me — and no one (including the patient) says thanks (p. 56).

Similarly, a majority of the husbands of mastectomy patients in a study by Maguire [15, p.495] reported that their adjustment was hindered by a 'lack of opportunity to talk to anyone about their worries'. Northouse [20] found that husbands of mastectomy patients perceived little support from physicians and nurses during their wives' hospitalization and after their wives returned home. In the terminal phase of cancer, spouses report that family and friends often grow tired of visiting and that physicians and nurses may leave the patient and spouse on their own to cope with the stress of the illness [9].

The research reviewed in the first section of the chapter suggests that cancer can have a stressful impact on family members. They report distress levels comparable to patients and experience the stressful effects of illness over an extended period of time.

Cancer and Intrafamily Relations

Not only does cancer have a stressful impact on family members as individuals, but it also affects family roles and relationships. Specifically, this section addresses how cancer affects the spouse dyad, the children, and the family's roles and priorities.

Impact on the Spouse Dyad

The family system is comprised of a series of subsystems that enable the family to carry out its primary function — supporting its members [3]. The spouse subsystem plays an integral role in providing support to spouses and in enabling them to adapt to stress. The spouse subsystem provides each spouse with a refuge from the demands of life and a resource for coping with internal and external stressors affecting the family [3].

Investigators have tried to determine what effect cancer has on the relationship between spouses. Lichtman [21] studied the impact of breast cancer on 78 patients, their significant others and their marital relationships. Contrary to the popular myth that breast cancer can cause the breakup of marriages, Lichtman found that only 7% of the marriages were dissolved following the diagnosis and treatment of breast cancer. Of the couples that separated, in only two cases was the separation attributed to the effects of the breast cancer. Typically, couples who reported that their marriages were satisfying prior to cancer also reported that their marriages were satisfying following the cancer diagnosis. Similarly, Lieber et al. [22] found that the stress of cancer did not produce marital breakups or emotional alienation among marital partners. Rather, feelings of affection toward one another either increased or remained unchanged.

While cancer does not appear to alter marital relationships appreciably, Chekryn [8] found that it can cause strains in marital relations, especially for couples dealing with recurrent cancer. Among the factors contributing to marital tensions were the repeated recurrence of the cancer, separations induced by hospitalization, role strain, and physical and psychological withdrawal on the part of the patient.

What impact does cancer have on couples' sexual behaviors? This question has been of concern primarily to investigators working with breast cancer patients and their husbands. Wellisch et al. [4] reported that sexuality and intimacy were altered following a mastectomy. Approximately 36% of the husbands reported that the mastectomy had a 'bad' or 'somewhat bad' influence on their sexual relationships. Typically, husbands who reported more sexual problems after the mastectomy also reported lower sexual satisfaction prior to the surgery. In the study by Maguire [15], one year after the wives' mastectomies, 29% of the husbands reported moderate to severe sexual difficulties. In Lichtman's [21] study, 25% of the husbands reported a decrease in sexual intercourse and 14% reported a decrease in affectionate behaviors.

In a study which did not focus exclusively on breast cancer, Leiber et al. [22] interviewed spouses and patients with advanced cancer to determine if their sexual needs or affectional needs changed during the course of cancer treatment. The majority of subjects reported a desire for more nonsexual physical closeness after the onset of cancer. There was not a concurrent increase in desire for intercourse. Only 6% of the individuals reported a desire for more sexual intercourse, whereas 37.5% reported a decreased desire for sexual intercourse. For the individuals interviewed in this study, needs for closeness were manifested through comforting gestures and reassurance.

Aside from marital and sexual strains, problems of communicating about cancer have been reported by couples during all phases of the illness. In the early diagnostic and treatment phase, Jamison et al. [23] found that 89% of the patients reported little or no discussion of emotional concerns with their spouse before surgery, 87% reported maintaining little discussion while in the hospital, and 50% reported continuing this pattern of little or no discussion at home. In the recurrent phase of illness, Chekryn [8] found that couples seldom talked about cancer recurrence or only discussed it to a limited degree. In the terminal phase of cancer, couples' difficulty discussing the illness and impending death have been reported by a number of investigators [9, 10, 24]. Estimates indicate that approximately 60–78% of the couples never discussed death with their partner [10, 24].

One factor that may contribute to communication difficulties is that spouses differ regarding how much they want to communicate about the illness. One partner may have a high need to discuss the illness while the other may have little need or no desire to discuss the illness. For example, Lichtman [21] found that mastectomy patients had a greater need than their husbands to discuss fears about recurrence. Husbands seldom wanted to discuss fears primarily because they thought that talking about recurrence might create negative emotions within their wives and either hinder their wives' adjustments or cause their cancer to recur. Overall, 22% of the women in Lichtman's study reported frustration at their husbands' limited communication with them about their concerns.

How important is it for couples to openly discuss their feelings about cancer? The reports are mixed. Favoring open communication, investigators have found that open communication with one's mate was a significant predictor of couples' marital adjustment following breast cancer [21]. In addition, higher levels of family expressiveness have been associated with better adjustment for mastectomy patients and their husbands [13, 20]. More effective communication has also been associated with better negotiation of altered family roles following a cancer diagnosis [25] and better adjustment of family members to bereavement [26].

However, some reports indicate that open communication is not the panacea for every couple coping with cancer. For example, 59% of the widows in one study who reported that they had not discussed death with their husbands, said that it made no difference in their adjustment [9]. In addition, some family members have reported that the 'secret to their success was that they never discussed cancer at all' [27]. For these family members, limited communication represented a strategic choice rather than an inability to communicate. It appears that the degree to which open communication will assist couples depends the couple's pre-illness communication patterns and each partner's unique communication preferences.

Impact on the Children

Although children are an integral part of the family system, little attention has been given to the impact of cancer on their lives. The lack of research in this area is not surprising since for years children have been treated as tangential to or even excluded from the patient's treatment plans. Nevertheless, a few studies have described the impact of cancer on children of adult cancer patients.

Buckley [28] conducted a study of 40 families in which one of the parents had advanced cancer and found that children's behavior problems increased by 33% during the parent's illness. Behavior problems reported included difficulties at school, sleep and eating disturbances, increased aggression, trouble relating to peers and antisocial behavior such as stealing. Lichtman et al. [29] found that approximately 25% of the children of breast cancer patients had adjustment problems related to their mother's cancer. In the same sample, 12% of the mothers reported that deterioration occurred in their relationships with their children.

Some investigators have found that the reactions of children vary according to the developmental stage of the child [30]. In children between the ages of 7 and 10, Lewis et al. [30] found that feelings of sadness, worry, and loneliness were common. Children at this age expressed concern about the safety of their family and wondered if the cancer would return. In children between 10 and 13 years, the investigators found that children's concerns centered on the disruption and change the parents's cancer caused for them. Children in this age group felt the need to take on more responsibility and to help more at home. In the adolescent aged group, investigators found that children had conflicting feelings — wanting to be with the ill parent but at the same time wanting to separate from the ill parent so that they could 'do their own thing' [30, p. 209]. Other investigators have reported acting-out behavior [18, 31] as well as rejecting behavior [29] in adolescents whose parents have cancer. Developmentally, the adolescent age group appears at especially high risk of experiencing behavioral problems following the parent's cancer.

While the reactions of children may vary according to their developmental stage, some reports indicate that children's reactions vary according to the child's gender-relationship to the parent. Lichtman et al. [29] found that women with breast cancer had significantly more problems in their relationships with their daughters than with their sons. Problems with daughters were of a greater magnitude and were characterized by rejection of the mother, defensiveness, argumentativeness, and acting distant toward the mother. The tumultuous nature of daughters' reactions to their mothers' mastectomies has been attributed to a number of factors such as the daughter's fear that she will inherit the disease [15, 29, 32], the rivalry between mother and daughter [31], and the high degree of support that mothers expect from daughters (rather than sons) following the cancer diagnosis [29].

Although adjustment difficulties have been reported in approximately 25–30% of children [28, 29], a sizeable number of parents have reported no changes or changes for the better following the parent's diagnosis of cancer. Among the positive outcomes reported have been that cancer has brought families closer together [18, 30], illness has increased understanding among family members [29], and the experience has fostered more quality time for family activities [30].

Some factors place children of cancer patients at higher risk than others. One factor appears to be the adjustment level of the parent with cancer. Buckley [28] found that when parents adjusted poorly to their cancer diagnoses, their children also adjusted poorly. Lichtman et al. [29] found that parents with lower adjustment scores reported more negative changes in parent-child relationships following the cancer diagnosis. Investigators have speculated that parents with poorer adjustment may either view their children's behavior more negatively or else behave in ways that drive their children away. Other speculation suggests the reverse — children's behavioral problems heighten the parents' difficulty of coping with the cancer [29].

Various disease and treatment characteristics of the parent's illness have also been linked to poorer adjustment in children. The longer the duration of the parent's illness the greater the number of behavioral problems reported in the children [28]. In addition, poorer diagnoses and more extensive surgeries have been associated with more problems in parent-child relationships [29].

Due to the paucity of research on the impact of cancer on children, several questions remain unanswered. For example, how is the parent's cancer diagnosis best discussed with children at different ages? How much information should children be given about their parent's illness? What promotes healthy disclosure about cancer? Does greater involvement of children in health education programs foster better adjustment? Clearly more research is needed in these areas. In addition, more data need to be obtained from the children rather than from parents about their children's actual feelings and experiences.

Impact on Family Roles and Priorities

Since the family system is comprised of a group of interrelated members, changes that affect one family member are often accompanied by changes in other family members [3]. Illnesses, such as cancer, can overload the coping mechanisms of family members who frequently need to take on additional roles of the ill member.

In a study of spouses of newly diagnosed cancer patients, Oberst and James [7] found that life-style disruption was a concern for over 50% of the spouses. Spouses reported that their employment and household schedules were altered, arrangements for child care changed, and social activities were curtailed. Frequent travel to and from the hospital for the patient's treatment was particularly problematic for spouses. Family members reported that alterations in their life-style usually lasted for approximately 3 months.

Role alterations are also reported by spouses of patients with advanced cancer. Gotay [19] found that patients with advanced cancer and their spouses were often very restricted in their activities. Spouses often needed to take on more of the patient's roles due to the patient's lack of energy or problems with mobility [19]. Welch [5] found that frequent rehospitalizations of the patient with recurrent cancer altered the mate's work role and even led to the mates being concerned about losing their jobs.

To determine if there were certain factors that assisted families with the role disruption following a cancer diagnosis, Vess et al. [25, 33] examined the role functioning of 54 families coping with cancer. Subjects were interviewed just after the initial diagnosis and again 5 months later. The investigators found that families that allocated responsibilities using achieved roles (i.e. according to members' abilities) rather than ascribed roles (i.e. according to stereotypic expectations) exhibited more family cohesion and less role strain. In addition, families who used open communication patterns appeared to be more effective in negotiating the alterations in family roles just after the diagnosis and 5 months later. Families with young children appeared to be at greater risk of developing role allocation problems. In these families, children were not old enough to take on primary family roles and the demands of child care added to the role overload of the healthy spouse [25].

Although cancer can create role disruptions within a family, it can also create a change in family priorities, a change that is often viewed positively by many family members. For example, Lovejoy [6] found that some family members decided to retire early, or quit their jobs, or placed elderly parents in nursing homes so that they could attend more to the ill family member. In a study of lung cancer patients and their spouses, Cooper [18] found that the majority of subjects acknowledged that their values had changed since the cancer diagnosis. She found that both patients and spouses became less interested in money matters and trivia and more interested in spending time with one another.

As discussed in this section, cancer has a significant impact on the intrafamily system. The spouse dyad, children, and family roles and priorities can all be affected. The research underscores the importance of utilizing clinical assessment models that have a family focus. The use of a family assessment will allow clinicians to identify the ripple effects of cancer on the entire family system.

Cancer and Family Caregiving Responsibilities

Increasingly, family members are being asked to assume the role of primary caregiver to the ill family member. While this is not a new expectation, the demands surrounding the caregiving role have changed. For example, patients are leaving acute care settings 'quicker and sicker'. This means that family members must provide more complex care earlier in the course of recovery. In addition, many cancer treatments, such as chemotherapy, are now routinely given in outpatient or home settings, leaving family members essentially on their own to manage the adverse side effects or complications.

While health care has been changing, today's families have been changing too. More dual-worker households and single-parent households, greater geographical dispersion of extended family members, and a decrease in family size have resulted in fewer family resources and less family time to take on growing health care responsibilities. The nature of the caregiving role and the home care needs reported by family members in this changing environment must be examined.

Nature of the Caregiving Role

Providing care to an ill family member is no easy task. Approximately 63% of the family members in Welch's study [5] said that they encountered difficulties providing care in the home. In a study of caregivers, Holing [16] found that approximately 43% of the family members said they had difficulty providing care to the ill member. Among the problems reported were: trying to lift or move a physically incapacitated family member, watching a family member experience physical symptoms, coping with emotional problems of the patient, and coping with their own exhaustion in providing care.

The caregiving role is especially difficult because it is usually continuous, day and night, 7 days a week. In addition, the endless demands of the role can keep the caregiver confined to the home. Even though caregivers in one study would have liked time away, they feared leaving the patient alone and often had no one whom they could call on to stay with the patient [5]. Because of the ongoing demands of the role, a number of investigators have also found that caregivers have problems getting enough sleep [5, 16, 34]. For example, Rose [35] found that a majority of family members caring for a terminally ill member reported difficulty sleeping because they were too worried to sleep (afraid the patient might die) or they needed to provide care to the ill member at night.

Caregivers often experience feelings of insecurity as well [17]. Some families lack information on how to provide physical care for the patient and are also unsure about how to handle emotional problems such as depression [10]. Some family members question if they are doing enough and feel guilty when mishaps occur, such as a patient failing [16]. Not knowing how to perform a specific procedure also adds to the caregiver's insecurity. As one family member so clearly described [16, p. 34]:

> The first time they sent him home, I was scared to death — I had to change the bag and the odor was horrible and I thought 'How am I going to do this?'

Family members report that the emotional energy associated with providing care outweighs the physical energy required [16].

It would be ideal if the family member assuming the caregiving role were in excellent physical health and had few other concurrent responsibilities. Unfortunately, that is not typically the case. Caregivers, like patients, are frequently older and have their own health problems. In a small study of caregivers, Googe and Varricchio [34] found that over half reported that their own health was unsatisfactory. In addition, some caregivers were also trying to manage household responsibilities and care for children. Although they received some assistance during the daytime, the caregivers reported that they seldom had help during the night.

Home Care Needs of Family Members

Given the demands of the caregiving role, what specific learning needs do family members report? Hind [17] interviewed 83 family members of patients with a variety of different kinds of cancer and found that family members needed guidance in the following areas: (1) understanding the patient's disease; (2) knowing what to expect in providing home care; (3) giving reassurance to the patient; (4) managing side effects of treatments; (5) giving injections, and (6) managing dietary needs.

Other investigators have reported that family members' learning needs are primarily in the physical aspects of care. For example, family members of advanced cancer patients said they wanted more information about comfort and pain management, ambulation, bowel management, skin care and wound care [36]. Family members also mentioned that they needed instruction in areas that require more judgment and knowledge, such as pain control or preparing special foods [35]. This emphasis on physical aspects of care is not surprising, because family members are not accustomed to providing complex aspects of care that used to be provided by health professionals in acute care settings.

Even though family members have learning needs, systematic methods of educating family members have not always been in place. Many family members reported that they most frequently learned new caregiving skills by trial and error, a method accompanied by a high degree of dissatisfaction by family members [36]. Very few family members learned skills from health personnel. Health professionals seldom provided follow-up visits to ensure that caregiving skills were properly carried out. In Hind's study [17] 27% of the family members reported the need for guidance with physical care, but only 12% stated that they received it. Other resource problems reported by family caregivers were limited accessibility to medical services [9] and lack of awareness of community resources [17, 35].

With the growing trend toward home health care, it is likely that more services will be available to family caregivers in the futue. There is some indication that these services may enhance family resources. For example, Edstrom and Miller [37] offered a home care course to a small number of family members that included content on nutrition, range of motion, comfort measures, and community resources. Although the evaluation of their program was limited, family members who participated in the course reported increased knowledge of community resources as well as increased feelings of capability to provide home care.

In general, studies on the caregiving role indicate that family members have specific needs for information or assistance in order to provide care to the ill member. These studies also suggest that professional assistance provided through home care agencies or planned educational courses may be helpful to these families. Studies on the learning needs of family members also point out that the major responsibility for the care of the ill member rests with the family, once again highlighting the vital but vulnerable position of the family.

Cancer and Family-Professional Relationships

The family-professional relationship is becoming more important as patients and family members cope with the effects of cancer. Professionals are beginning to realize that they need a stronger alliance with family members to facilitate effectively the family members' primary caregiving responsibilities. This section discusses the nature of the family-professional relationship, family members' needs for access to information, and helpful professional behaviors identified by family members.

Nature of the Relationships

In busy health care settings, health professionals have little time to develop effective interpersonal relationships with family members. Typically, contacts between health professional and family members are quite limited. Krant and Johnston [10] interviewed 126 family members of cancer patients and found that 78% of the family members reported either no contact or a little contact with physicians. Only 9% reported that they were able to talk freely with physicians. Similar findings were reported by Bond [38, 39] who found that the majority of family members reported no contact with physicians or nurses. In the few instances in which interactions did occur, the contact between health professionals and family members was typically a single meeting that occurred by chance and was initiated by family members.

There are several reasons why the contact among professionals and family members is so limited [40]. First, family members and physicians are seldom in the hospital at the same time. Physicians frequently make rounds early in the morning, while family members visit patients in the afternoon or evening. This leaves little opportunity for informal contact among professionals and family members. Second, the responsibility for initiating the interaction appears to rest on family members, who are often hesitant to bother busy physicians and nurses. Professionals tend not to initiate interactions unless there is a change in the medical status of the patient [38, 39]. Third, both professionals and family members tend to see their relationship as less important than the professional-patient relationship. Family members repeatedly prioritize their own needs lower than patient needs [41, 42] and often do not expect help from professionals [43].

What effect does limited contact have on professional-family relationships? There is some evidence to suggest that when initial contact is limited, it can hinder the development of long-term professional-family relationships. Krant and Johnston [10] found, for example, that family members who did not have an initial discussion with the physician said they were reluctant to talk with the physician later on. Another problem with limited contact is that family members do not have direct access to information, but must rely on secondary sources or 'filtered communication' which is less accurate than direct communication [44]. Furthermore, limited contact prevents the development of a supportive relationship that could buffer the stress experienced by family members. Given the limited contact with professionals reported by family members in one study, it is not surprising that only 33% of the family members found the physician to be of help to the family [10].

Access to Information

Even though professional contact with families may be limited, family members of cancer patients have a high need for information from professionals. From a list of need statements, Wright and Dyck [45] found that family members of hospitalized cancer patients gave the highest ratings to the need to be kept informed of the patients's condition. Similarly, Tringali [46] found that the need to have questions answered honestly was rated the highest by family members across all phases of illness.

Although family members place a high priority on obtaining accurate information, they report considerable difficulty actually getting information. Forty-nine percent of the family members in a study by Wright and Dyck [45] mentioned difficulty getting information. Specific problems included getting concrete answers from physicians, getting in touch with physicians, obtaining information via the telephone, and getting information about the patient's daily progress from nurses. Family members also report a lack of availability of health professionals and the lack of private settings in which to obtain information [39].

Family members often view health professionals as controllers of information [47]. A study of family members of patients receiving palliative care identified the following ways that professionals controlled information: 'How questions were answered, the extent to which explanations were offered, the degree to which health professionals would interpret facts, and how available they were to families and patients' [47].

Control of information also extends to which health care professionals can give family members information. The physician is often seen as the legitimate provider of information. Some family members are hesitant to ask nurses for diagnostic and treatment information since family members believe that nurses are restricted in the amount and type of information that they can give [39, 43, 48]. Overall, family members' access to information becomes limited when physicians are not accessible and when other professionals such as nurses are not viewed as legitimate sources of information.

Helpful Professional Behaviors

What can health professionals do that would be particularly helpful to family members of cancer patients? Lovejoy [6] asked 105 family members of hospitalized cancer patients to describe the ways in which nurses helped them. Family members' responses were categorized into three areas. The first area, validation of worth, referred to a nurses's behavior that confirmed the personal value of the family member, such as showing respect, listening to family members, being responsive, and conveying an attitude to the family that 'we're in this together' [6, p. 36]. The second area, providing assurance, referred to nurses' behaviors that reduced family members' uncertainty, such as demonstrating professional competence, projecting a positive attitude, and anticipating family members' needs. The third area of behaviors, called preparation for the unknown, referred to behaviors which reduced the strangeness of new situations — such as keeping the family informed and orienting family members to new procedures.

In another study, family members of patients receiving palliative care identified 77 professional behaviors that were important to the care of the family [47]. Among the most frequently reported behaviors were: including the family in conversations with the patient, providing the family with information, being available to family members, listening to information provided by the family, treating the family in a friendly and polite manner, encouraging family members to ask for information, and providing straightforward answers to questions.

In highlighting the research on the relationships between professionals and family, the overriding issue appears to be that professionals need to establish contact with family members in a planned, systematic manner. Without that contact, professionals are not able to assess family members' reactions to the illness, much less provide information and support to family members.

Clinical Implications

Although the amount of research on the impact of cancer on the family is limited, several clinical implications emerge from a review of the research. The major implication is that clinical assessments of clients' psychosocial adjustment need to be family-focused rather than patient-focused. A broader family-based assessment will allow clinicians to identify the concurrent effects of the illness on family members as well as on patients. Ideally, family assessments should be conducted over an extended period of time because family members' needs vary over the course of illness.

There is a need to identify families that are at high risk of having adjustment problems following the patient's diagnosis. Since many family members adapt fairly well to the cancer experience without professional assistance [49], a high-risk profile would help professionals to allocate resources to families in particular need of professional assistance. Although there has not been enough research in this area to develop a profile of families at risk, the following factors have been associated with higher levels of family stress: family members perceiving little support [20], family members of patients receiving active treatment or palliative care [12], and spouses of patients who report high levels of stress [12, 13].

Since existing research indicates that between one third and one fourth of couples report sexual difficulties following the cancer diagnosis, it may be useful to assess whether or not changes have occurred in couples' sexual relationships. Assessment of couples' pre-cancer sexual functioning is important because couples with more sexual problems prior to the illness appear at higher risk of having difficulties after the illness. Furthermore, it may be useful to assess how couples communicate about the illness since partners' communication preferences may differ at times and may be a source of strain.

The research indicates that clinicians need to assess the reactions of children to their parents' cancer, because some studies find that approximately one third of the children will develop behavioral problems. Children of parents who have adjustment problems or a lingering illness may be at higher risk of developing their own adjustment difficulties. Adolescents of parents with cancer may be at risk due to the concurrent developmental turmoil they are experiencing.

Special attention also needs to be directed to families that are giving complex care to the ill member at home. Adequate discharge teaching needs to be given to both patients and family members. Family members need to acquire skills and information that will enhance their ability and sense of competence. Professionals also need to establish an ongoing mechanism for maintaining follow-up with family caregivers.

Finally, the research reviewed in this chapter underscores the importance of maintaining effective family-professional relationships. Family members have needs for direct, understandable information from health professionals. In addition, family members need to give as well as receive information; they want to be treated as integral members of the health care team. Greater attention to family issues in cancer care will enable both patients and family members to cope with the effects of cancer.

References

1 Cassileth, B.; Hamilton, J.: The famly with cancer; in Cassileth, The cancer patient (Lea & Febiger, Philadelphia 1979).

2 Bowen, M. family reaction to death; in Guerin, Family therapy (Gardner Press, New York 1976).

3 Minuchin, S.: Families and family therapy (Harvard University Press, Cambridge 1974).

4 Wellisch, D.K.; Jamison, K.R.; Pasnau, R.O.: Psychological aspects of mastectomy. II. The man's perspective. Am. J. Psychiat. *135:* 543–546 (1978).

5 Welch, D.: Planning nursing interventions for family members of adult cancer patients. Cancer Nurs. *4:* 365–370 (1981).

6 Lovejoy, N.C.: Family responses to cancer hospitalization. Oncol. Nurs. Forum *2:* 33–37 (1986).

7 Oberst, M. James, R.H.: Going home: patient and spouse adjustment following cancer surgery. Top. clin. Nurs. *7:* 46–57 (1985).

8 Chekryn, J.: Cancer recurrence: personal meaning, communication and marital adjustment. Cancer Nurs. *7:* 491–498 (1984).

9 Vachon, M.L.; Freedman, K.; Formo, A.; et al.: The final illness in cancer: the widow's perspective. Can. med. Ass. J. *117:* 1151–1153 (1977).

10 Krant, M.J. Johnston, L.: Family members' perception of communication in late stage cancer. Int. J. Psychiat. Med. *8:* 203–216 (1977–1978).

11 Northouse, L.L.; Swain, J.A.: Adjustment of patients and husbands to the initial impact of breast cancer. Nursing Res. *36:* 221–225 (1987).

12 Cassileth, B.; Lusk, E.J.; Strouse, T.B.; et al.: A psychological analysis of cancer patients and their next-of-kin. Cancer *55:* 72–76 (1985).

13 Baider, L.; Kaplan De-Nour, A.: Couples' reactions and adjustment to mastectomy: a preliminary report. Int. J. Psychiat. Med. *14:* 265–276 (1984).

14 Plumb, M.M.; Holland, J.: Comparative studies of psychological function in patients with advanced cancer. I. Self-reported depressive symptoms. Psychosom. Med. *39:* 264–291 (1977).

15 Maguire, P.: The repercussions of mastectomy on the family. Int. J. Fam. Psychiat. *1:* 485–503 (1981).

16 Holing, E.V.: The primary caregivers perception of the dying trajectory. Cancer Nurs. *9:* 29–37 (1986).
17 Hinds, C.: The needs of families who care for patients with cancer at home: are we meeting them? J. Adv. Nurs. *10:* 575–581 (1985).
18 Cooper, E.T.: A pilot study on the effects of the diagnosis of lung cancer on family relationships. Cancer Nurs. *7:* 301–308 (1984).
19 Gotay, C.C.: The experience of cancer during early and advanced stages: the views of patients and their mates. Soc. Sci. Med. *18:* 605–613 (1984).
20 Northouse, L.L.: The role of social support in the adjustment of patients and husbands to breast cancer. Nursing Res. (in press).
21 Lichtman, R.: Close relationships after breast cancer; unpubl. doct. diss., Los Angeles (1982).
22 Leiber, L.; Plumb, M.M.; Gerstenzang, M.L.; Holland, J.: The communication of affection between cancer patients and their spouses. Psychosom. Med. *38:* 379–388 (1976).
23 Jamison, K.R.; Wellisch, D.K.; Pasnau, R.O.: Psychosocial aspects of mastectomy. I. The woman's perspective. Am. J. Psychiat. *135:* 432–436 (1978).
24 Hinton, J.: Sharing or withholding awareness of dying between husband and wife. J. psychosom. Res. *25:* 337–343 (1981).
25 Vess, J.D.; Moreland, J.R.; Schwebel, A.I.: An empirical assessment of the effects of cancer on famly role functioning. J. psychosol. Oncol. *3:* 1–16 (1985).
26 Cohen, P.; Dizenhuz, I.M.; Winget, C.: Family adaptation to terminal illness and death of a parent. Soc. Casework *58:* 223–228 (1977).
27 Thorne, S.: The family experience. Cancer Nurs. *8:* 223–228 (1977).
28 Buckley, I.E.: Listen to the children: impact on the mental health of children of a parent's catastrophic illness (Cancer Care, New York 1977).
29 Lichtman, R.R.; Taylor, S.E.; Wood, J.V. et al.: Relations with children after breast cancer: the mother-daughter relationship at risk. J. psychosol. Oncol. *2:* 1–19 (1984).
30 Lewis, F.M.; Ellison, E.S.; Woods, N.F.: The impact of breast cancer on the family. Semin. Oncol. Nurs. *1:* 206–213 (1985).
31 Wellisch, D.K.: Family relationships of the mastectomy patient: interactions with the spouse and children. Israel J. med. Scis *17:* 993–996 (1981!.
32 Grandsraff, N.W.: The impact of breast cancer on the family. Front. Radiat. Ther. Onc., vol. 11, pp. 146–156 (Karger, Basel 1976).
33 Vess, J.D.; Moreland, J.R.; Schwebel, A.J.: A follow-up study of role functioning and the psychological environment of the family of cancer patients. J. psychosoc. Oncol. *3:* 1–14 (1985).
34 Googe, M.C.; Varricchio, C.: A pilot investigation of home health care needs of cancer patients and their families. Oncol. Nursing Forum *8:* 24–28 (1981).
35 Rose, M.A.: Problems families face in home care. Am. J. Nurs. *76* 416–418 (1976).
36 Grobe, M.F. Ilstrup, D.M.; Ahmann, D.J.: Skills needed by family members to maintain the care of an advanced cancer patient. Cancer Nurs. *4:* 371–375 (1981).
37 Edstrom, S.; Miller, M.W.: Preparing the family to care for the cancer patient at home: a home care course. Cancer Nurs. *4:* 49–52 (1981).
38 Bond, S.: Communicating with families of cancer patients. 1. The relatives and doctors. Nursing Times *78:* 962–965 (1982).
39 Bond, S.: Communicating with families of cancer patients. 2. The nurses. Nursing Times *78:* 1027–1029 (1982).

40 Northouse, P.G. Northouse, L.L.: Communication and cancer: issues confronting patients, health professionals, and family members. J. psychosoc. Oncol. *5:* 15–41 (1987).

41 Freihofer, P.; Felton, G.: Nursing behaviors in bereavement. Nursing Res. *25:* 332–337 (1976).

42 Skorupka, P.; Bohnet, N.: Primary caregivers' perceptions of nursing behaviors that best meet their needs in a home care hospice setting. Cancer Nurs. *5:* 371–374 (1982).

43 Hampe, S.: Needs of the grieving spouse in a hospital setting. Nursing Res. *24:* 113–120 (1975).

44 Northouse, P.G.; Northouse, L.L.: Health commmunication: a handbook for health professionals (Prentice-Hall, Englewood Cliffs 1985).

45 Wright, K.; Dyck, S.: Expressed concerns of adult cancer patients' family members. Cancer Nurs. *7:* 371–374 (1984).

46 Tringali, C.: The needs of family members of cancer patients. Oncol. Nursing Forum *13:* 65–70 (1986).

47 Kristjanson, L.: Indicators of quality of palliative care from a family perspective. J. palliat. Care *1:* 8–17 (1986).

48 Dyck, S.; Wright, K.: Family perceptions: the role of the nurse throughout an adult's cancer experience. Oncol. Nursing Forum *12:* 53–56 (1986).

49 Goldberg, R.J.; Wool, M.: Psychotherapy for the spouses of lung cancer patients: assessment of an intervention. Psychother. Psychosom. *43:* 141–150 (1985).

Laurel L. Northouse, PhD, RN, College of Nursing,
Wayne State University, 5557 Cass, Detroit, MI 48202 (USA)

Adv. psychosom. Med., vol. 18, pp. 102–118 (Karger, Basel 1988)

The Role of Concrete Services in Cancer Care[1]

Vincent Mor[a], *Edward Guadagnoli*[a], *Margaret Wool*[b]

[a]Brown University, Center for Health Care Research, Providence, R.I.;
[b]Rhode Island Hospital, Department of Psychiatry, Providence, R.I., USA

Introduction

The scope and nature of cancer treatment in the USA is experiencing a significant transformation. Additionally, the prevalence of individuals undergoing cancer treatment is increasing rapidly. The aging of the general population translates into further growth in the number of persons with the disease [1–4]. With the trend toward earlier identification of cancer, patients face longer periods of survival post-diagnosis, with persistent symptoms and increased use of oncological treatment services [5–7].

In addition to an increase in the number of cancer patients, there has also been a recent augmentation in the number of practicing cancer specialists. Federal training support and the outreach of Cooperative Groups to community practitioners has led to a proliferation of oncologists, and thus, more patients receiving specialty care.

Treatment successes with leukemia, using intensive chemotherapeutic interventions, have been applied to solid tumors with some success in breast and testicular cancers. At the same time, the trend toward the 'dehospitalization' of medical treatment has begun to reach oncology as it has other disciplines [8]. Extended outpatient care, surgi-centers, same-day administration of invasive diagnostic procedures, day hospital administration of complex chemotherapy and associated treatments, along with the trend to administer these regimens at home are all testimony to the movement away from the acute hospital as the locus of care [9–18].

[1] This work was supported in part by Grant Number CA 41020 from the National Cancer Institute.

The net effect of increased cancer prevalence and 'dehospitalization' is more people receiving aggressive care outside the protective environment of the hospital. Patients' needs for various forms of assistance and support are exacerbated by disease progression and the toxic side effects of the treatments received [19, 22].

Assistance at home may become necessary as a result of patients' inability to meet their own daily living and treatment-related needs [19–21]. In the past, such patients would have spent more time under the care of nurses in the hospital. With recent changes in health service reimbursement and delivery, patients are being discharged 'quicker and sicker' to recuperate at home. The capacity of the community support system to meet the demands of patients undergoing long-term cancer treatment is an important issue with current and future implications.

Traditionally, needs have been met by families organizing a system of informal care. However, with the increasing complexity of intensive treatments performed on an outpatient basis or at home, and with the changing composition of the American family (in 1983, 23 million persons lived alone or with unrelated persons [23]), the role of the formal home care system is likely to become increasingly important if the trend toward community-based treatment is to continue. Consequently, clinicians working with cancer patients and their families must be cognizant of both the burden that caretaking imposes, as well as the confusion engendered as they struggle through complex bureaucratic and insurance hurdles to secure needed formal services.

The intent of this chapter is to survey the prevalence of concrete service needs (such as personal care, meal preparation, child care, shopping, housekeeping, transportation, and financial assistance), and to examine variables associated with the intensity of met and unmet need. The findings of these analyses are discussed in terms of their implications for clinical intervention with cancer patients. Particular attention is paid to the interface between concrete needs and the appearance of emotional adjustment and/or psychiatric problems. It is the goal of this chapter to underscore the importance of concrete needs in patients' and families' adjustment to cancer. This material is also designed to encourage psychiatric clinicians to become more flexible in departing from a strictly medical model to consider important adaptational aspects of their patients' experience. Such an approach will enhance the cancer caregiver's capacity to resolve many patient complaints which do not respond to 'symptom management' in the traditional sense.

Defining Needs and Problems

Until recently, the major focus of research on cancer patients' needs has been in the psychological domain [24–26]. However, reports are appearing in the literature regarding patients' problems with functioning in their community after or during treatment [27–29]. The hospice movement also stimulated numerous authors to describe the needs of patients and their families as they approached the terminal phase of their illness [30, 31]. Over the disease course, patients' need for concrete services is predictable. As patients' independent functioning wanes, their need for assistance increases. Needs may also result from the bureaucratic complications, financial burdens, and emotional stresses which often accompany the onset and course of a major illness.

Bureaucratic complications arise as patients and their families try to interact with service agencies. Financial deprivations accumulate as out-of-pocket expenditures for insurance deductibles and copayments are required, medication costs increase, and as income losses due to sickness have a growing impact on family financial resources. In addition, the disease and its consequences carry an emotional burden, which is an ongoing fact of life-threatening illness and the effect of illness on patients' and families' lifestyles.

Cancer patients' needs arise in different domains of life functioning. One way to avoid the 'laundry list' approach of enumerating needs, which characterizes much of the literature [19], is to group needs into personal care, instrumental/household, and administrative domains as has been advocated in gerontology [32]. Personal care refers to activities such as dressing and bathing. Instrumental activities comprise shopping, cooking, and cleaning, while administrative needs include identifying and securing diverse pieces of information and services ranging from medical appliance acquisition and consumable medical supplies to advocacy with insurance companies. Uncontrolled symptoms may lead to impaired function but also represent a distinct area of need for medical intervention. Disease progression and active treatment can reduce the individual's ability to meet these needs independently. Additionally, the feelings of dependence generated by having others perform these functions may, in some instances, lead to emotional adjustment problems.

Fortunately for the purposes of understanding the problems faced by cancer patients and families, whether defined as needs and unresolved symptoms or specified in terms of diverse problems, there seems to be a substantial correlation between both the number of problems and the number of needs experienced. Using the approach of reviewing domains of needs makes it possible to differentiate between met and unmet needs. *Unmet* needs are areas in which the patient requires assistance but for which help is not forthcoming or is insufficient [19].

The authors reviewed the available literature regarding the prevalence of cancer patients' needs or problems. In recognition of the multidimensional character of patients' concrete needs [33], the disparate array of needs was categorized into the major dimensions of need — Physical, Instrumental, and Administrative — as suggested by Pfeiffer [32]. Table I presents data abstracted from 12 different studies of cancer patients. The footnotes briefly describe each sample in terms of disease progression as well as the mode of data collection and need estimate. The studies were displayed so that samples presented were in order of increasing progression of disease, identified, respectively, by higher Roman numerals in the table heading.

Despite the differences in samples, the data suggest that cancer patients' needs increase with the severity or duration of disease. For example, studies IX, X, and XI document the terminal patient's increased need for services and the increased demands placed upon family members [28, 30]. Newly diagnosed patients' needs (IIb), however, are substantially lower [34]. The positive correlation between disease progression and need is apparent for the personal and instrumental need dimensions. A similar relationship was observed in a life study of 246 breast cancer patients undergoing treatment. Selby et al. [35] found that patients with metastatic progression manifested greater impairment than did patients receiving adjuvant chemotherapy. Patients with metastatic disease were more impaired in areas of mobility, breathing, pain, physical activity, housework, writing, and appetite. While some authors have suggested that cancer type might also affect the level of need, it is likely that this finding is attributable to different rates of disease progression in the different cancers [35, 36].

Demographic factors have also been reported to influence the presence of need. Older patients are more frail due to preexisting chronic diseases as has been reported by Craig et al. [37]. Among breast cancer patients, Feldman et al. [38] found that nonwhites were three times more likely to experience disability than were whites. The authors suggested that economic factors accounted for this differential finding, and recently Mor et al. [19] confirmed the effect of income on need across all dimensions.

With increasing debility, cancer patients generally rely upon their families for various types of assistance. Thus, the principal determinant of

Table I. Reported concrete needs (%)[1] of cancer patients by study

Need domain	Study											
	I[a]	IIa[b]	IIb[c]	III[d]	IV[e]	V[f]	VI[g]	VII[h]	VIII[i]	IX[j]	X[k]	XI[l]
Physical												
Ambulation	23						22		46			83
Transfer	7			25	32		8		29			
Eating				<1	31	63	21	50	16	25		
Sleeping					29	60						
Self-care				2	17	38		57		65		75
Pain	29				28	87	25					
Dressings		44	16		18							88
Instrumental												
Daily home help				14		61		53	77			
Home care nursing		22		4				47	64	70		
Transportation	7	7	16			47	5	60		38		
Shopping				4					53			
Meal prep.				3					51			
Equipment		29	16					63				
Child care	2			3			3	1				
Administrative												
Financial	20			6	11	48	16	43	19		13	13
Paperwork							4		21		31	43
Information							9		72			
Finding help									68		35	46

[1]Percentages are rounded to the nearest whole number.
[a]Lehmann et al. [36]: 805 randomly selected patients, heterogeneous with respect to cancer type and disease progression. Data collected through interview and chart review.
[b]Stengle and Eckert [34]; 708 colorectal cancer patients served by the Michigan Cancer Foundation (MCF) (1977–1981), heterogeneous with respect to disease progression. Service statistics reported.
[c]Stengle and Eckert [34]; newly diagnosed colorectal cancer patients served by MCF (January 1982 to September 1982). Service statistics reported.
[d]American Cancer Society [45]; 810 patients, heterogeneous with respect to cancer type and disease progression, asked what services were required at illness onset.
[e]Schomburg et al. [29]: 365 patients, heterogeneous with respect to cancer type and disease progression, undergoing treatment. Data collected through interview.
[f]Heinrich et al. [27]; 84 patients, heterogeneous with respect to cancer type and disease progression, undergoing treatment. Data collected through interview.
[g]Houts [47]; 631 patients, diagnosed within a 2-year period prior to interview, heterogeneous with respect to cancer type. Data collected through interview. Figures reported represent statewide estimates.

whether patients' needs are met is the presence of a resilient family-helping network. Whereas disease progression will predict how much help patients will need and the problems they experience, social factors are central to determining how well such needs will be met.

The remainder of this chapter will present data from a recently completed survey of cancer patients' needs undertaken by the authors as part of a research project funded by the National Cancer Institute (Grant No. CA 41020). Data presented relate to the prevalence of need by dimension and type of need and whether or not that need is met.

A Study of Cancer Treatment Patients' Concrete Service Needs

Patients undergoing chemotherapy were identified at two of Rhode Island's hospital-based oncology clinics and at eight of the state's 19 private oncology practices. A total of 413 patients were interviewed over the 6-month period beginning April 1986. Patients selected for study received treatment within one month of the survey and were 21 years of age or older.

Interviews took place only with the permission of patients' treating physicians. Physician refusals (2%) were extremely low. The refusal rate obtained for patients (22%) was within the 20–25% normally encountered in this type of data collection. Sex and treatment location (clinic versus private practice) distributions did not differ between patient refuser and nonrefuser groups. Patients who refused, however, tended to be older.

Table I (cont.)

[h]Grobe et al. [46]: 30 late-stage patients, heterogeneous with respect to cancer type. Data collected through interview.
[i]Mor et al. [19]; 217 late-stage, service agency patients, heterogeneous with respect to cancer type. Data collected through interview.
[j]Gold [28]; families of recently deceased patients, patients heterogeneous with respect to cancer type. Data collected through interview.
[k]Greer et al. (National Hospice Study) [30]; primary care persons of 297 terminal cancer nonhospice patients, heterogeneous with respect to cancer type. Data collected through interview.
[l]Greer et al. (National Hospice Study) [30]; primary care persons of 833 home care hospice patients, heterogeneous with respect to cancer type. Data collected through interview.

Most (47%) of the patients interviewed were diagnosed with breast cancer. This accounts for the large overall proportion (71%) of female patients in the sample. No other diagnosis predominated among remaining patients. Patient age, in this predominantly white sample, ranged from 21 to 91 (M = 60.37, SD = 13.65). The majority (63%) of patients received palliative care (affording relief, but not cure). Twenty-five percent of patients were receiving some form of adjuvant treatment, in which 'disease free' (post-surgical) patients are given prophylactic treatment. Oncological intervention for remaining patients was strictly curative in intent. The majority of patients (55%) were diagnosed over one year (M = 3.18, SD = 4.46) prior to interview.

The interview, performed over the telephone, contained items assessing physical functioning, general health, quality of life, financial status, presence of symptoms, and concrete service needs in each of the three need dimensions described earlier. For each need area or functional activity, patient need status was determined. *No need* was defined by independent performance; *met need* existed if patient received assistance and no additional assistance was needed; and need was *unmet* if the patient continued to require help or any additional help with the task. A similar coding scheme was employed for symptom status. Symptoms are defined as *relieved* if help was sought and some measure of relief was obtained. *Unrelieved* symptoms occurred when patients did not seek symptom relief or when relief was sought but not obtained.

Prevalence of Concrete Service Needs

The sample's need status is displayed in table II. Percentages are presented as a function of cancer type and aim of treatment (curative/adjuvant versus palliative). Data are presented for those patients (n = 405) for whom each of these variables was known. Given the large proportion of breast cancer patients in the sample and the absence of other homogeneous diagnostic groups, data are presented for breast and nonbreast cancer patients. Aim of treatment is used to contrast need because it is related to disease duration and to general functional status. Patients who receive palliative care are more likely to have had the disease for a longer time period and are often less functional.

Few patients reported either need or unmet need in the personal activities area (bathing or mobility; table II). Both of these activities have been shown to be the more difficult elements in the Activities of Daily Living hierarchy [39], meaning that most patients could perform other activities such as toileting and feeding. Overall, 14% of patients reported need in the personal area, while only 4% reported one or more unmet needs.

Instrumental activities provided more of a challenge to patients. Most patients (88%) reported need for help with at least one activity. Unmet need was reported by nearly one fifth (19%) of the sample. Examination of table II reveals that breast patients were more independent, for most activities, than were nonbreast patients. This is probably due to sex differences between groups. Males, who traditionally are less likely to perform these activities, are absent from the breast cancer group. Breast patients receiving palliative care generally reported both more need and unmet need than did other breast cancer patients. For nonbreast cancer patients, need levels were similar for palliative and nonpalliative patients within each activity. Unmet need, however, was generally greater for palliative patients. For both groups, need and unmet need were greatest for heavy housework. Levels of need and unmet need reported for home health care, chemotherapy home health care, and child care were very low compared to other activities. Although we asked about it, there were almost no patients who received chemotherapy at home. While apparently a growing phenomenon in some parts of the country, it has still not become popular in the Northeast.

The proportion of patients reporting need for help with administrative activities (44%) fell between the levels reported for personal and instrumental activities. Unmet need in at least one administrative activity was reported by 11% of the sample. Both breast and nonbreast patients required the greatest assistance with filling out forms. Independence levels for all activities were similar across patient groups. For both groups, obtaining information about one's disease or treatment yielded the greatest degree of unmet need.

Care Providers

Patients who reported receiving help with any type of activity were asked who provided assistance. Family members were reported to provide care most often (typically, in more than 75% of the cases) for the majority of activities. Service agency or professional personnel provided a large proportion of assistance (> 50%) with home health, financial, legal, and information needs. Assistance from friends was rarely reported.

When service agency or professional help was not received, either because other help was provided or because no help was required at that

Table II. Need status by cancer type and extent of disease

Domain	Breast		Nonbreast	
	curative/adjuvant n = 84	palliative n = 98	curative/adjuvant n = 58	palliative n = 155
Personal				
Bathing				
None	97.9	76.5	94.8	83.9
Met	1.1	17.3	5.2	12.9
Unmet	1.1	6.1	0.0	3.2
Mobility				
None	95.7	86.6	98.3	91.0
Met	0.0	10.3	1.7	7.7
Unmet	4.3	3.1	0.0	1.3
Instrumental				
Meal preparation				
None	73.4	63.3	33.3	32.1
Met	23.4	30.6	66.7	64.1
Unmet	3.2	6.1	0.0	3.8
Light house				
None	68.1	45.4	29.8	30.5
Met	24.5	44.3	64.9	61.7
Unmet	7.4	10.3	5.3	7.8
Heavy house				
None	40.4	23.7	17.5	15.5
Met	48.9	50.8	75.4	72.3
Unmet	10.6	15.5	7.0	12.3
Shopping				
None	59.6	32.0	21.4	23.1
Met	39.4	60.8	73.2	71.2
Unmet	1.1	7.2	5.4	5.8
Transportation to MD				
None	58.7	33.7	43.9	36.8
Met	38.0	58.2	54.4	57.4
Unmet	3.3	8.2	1.8	5.8
Other transportation				
None	78.7	41.8	66.7	53.8
Met	19.1	45.9	31.6	43.6
Unmet	2.1	12.2	1.8	2.6
Home health				
None	95.7	89.8	87.7	84.6
Met	4.3	10.2	12.3	14.1
Unmet	0.0	0.0	0.0	1.3

Table II. (cont.)

Chemo. home health				
None	100.0	99.0	98.2	99.4
Met	0.0	1.0	1.8	0.6
Unmet	0.0	0.0	0.0	0.0
Child care				
None	95.7	99.0	96.5	96.1
Met	4.3	1.0	1.8	1.9
Unmet	0.0	0.0	1.8	1.9
Administrative				
Forms				
None	72.3	62.9	70.7	65.4
Met	25.5	34.0	27.6	32.1
Unmet	2.1	3.1	1.7	2.6
Financial advice				
None	85.1	91.7	96.6	90.4
Met	10.6	6.3	3.4	5.8
Unmet	4.3	2.1	0.0	3.8
Legal advice				
None	95.7	93.8	89.7	91.7
Met	3.2	5.2	8.6	6.4
Unmet	1.1	1.0	1.7	1.9
Information about disease				
None	88.3	89.7	94.8	89.1
Met	3.2	3.1	5.2	3.2
Unmet	8.5	7.2	0.0	7.7

time, patients were asked if they knew of agencies that could provide help if needed. Within each need domain, the majority (> 55%) of patients reported that they did not know of any agencies that could provide help. When asked if they would consider using such services in the future, approximately 16% stated they would not seek agency help for either Personal, Instrumental, or Administrative needs.

Symptom Prevalence

The proportion of patients reporting selected symptoms and whether these symptoms were resolved is displayed in table III. For the total sample, most frequently reported symptoms were fatigue (68%), dry mouth (45%), pain (44%), and nausea (39%). Breast cancer patients receiving palliative treatment reported greater relieved and unrelieved symptom occurrence in

Table III. Symptom status by cancer type and extent of disease

Symptom	Breast		Nonbreast	
	curative/adjuvant n = 84	palliative n = 98	curative/adjuvant n = 58	palliative n = 155
Hair loss				
None	74.5	72.4	75.4	78.6
Met	13.8	10.2	7.0	5.2
Unmet	11.7	17.3	17.5	16.2
Pain				
None	69.1	42.3	60.3	54.2
Met	19.1	43.3	25.9	34.8
Unmet	11.7	14.4	13.8	11.0
Nausea				
None	63.8	60.8	57.9	61.3
Met	24.5	16.5	31.6	24.5
Unmet	11.7	22.7	10.5	14.2
Dry mouth				
None	67.7	51.5	56.9	46.8
Met	25.8	41.2	37.9	41.7
Unmet	6.5	7.2	5.2	11.5
Constipation				
None	80.9	71.1	77.6	77.3
Met	16.0	20.6	15.5	19.5
Unmet	3.2	8.2	6.9	3.2
Diarrhea				
None	88.3	83.3	82.8	73.1
Met	6.4	12.5	3.4	13.5
Unmet	5.3	4.2	13.8	13.5
Sore mouth				
None	89.4	91.7	79.3	84.0
Met	5.3	6.3	8.6	7.7
Unmet	5.3	2.1	12.0	8.3
Poor appetite				
None	83.0	70.8	65.0	52.6
Met	6.4	10.4	14.0	17.5
Unmet	10.6	18.8	21.1	29.9
Weight loss				
None	83.9	74.2	58.6	67.9
Met	1.1	3.1	10.3	7.7
Unmet	15.1	22.7	31.0	24.4
Sleep problems				
None	68.1	72.9	58.6	67.1
Met	8.5	11.5	20.7	16.1
Unmet	23.4	15.6	20.7	16.8

Table III. (cont.)

Weight gain				
None	76.6	77.9	67.2	75.0
Met	6.4	3.2	8.6	0.7
Unmet	17.0	18.9	24.1	24.3
Fatigue				
None	42.6	27.8	43.9	23.2
Met	41.5	47.4	36.8	49.0
Unmet	16.0	24.7	19.3	27.7
Bleeding				
None	93.5	88.7	93.1	91.7
Met	3.2	3.1	0.0	1.9
Unmet	3.2	8.2	6.9	6.4
Burning urination				
None	93.5	89.6	98.3	92.9
Met	3.2	8.3	1.7	3.2
Unmet	3.2	2.1	0.0	3.8
Fever				
None	93.6	94.7	91.4	91.7
Met	3.2	5.3	0.0	3.8
Unmet	3.2	0.0	8.6	4.5
Short breath				
None	76.3	60.8	79.3	64.9
Met	15.1	20.6	8.6	10.5
Unmet	8.6	18.6	12.1	15.6
Swelling				
None	77.4	69.8	89.7	80.5
Met	9.7	17.7	5.2	9.7
Unmet	12.9	12.5	5.2	9.7

the areas of pain, constipation, fatigue, and shortness of breath than did other patients. Fatigue, both relieved and unrelieved, occurred more frequently for nonbreast patients receiving palliative care than for those receiving treatment for adjuvant or curative purposes. Not surprisingly, approximately one fifth of the total sample reported unresolved poor appetite, weight loss, weight gain, and fatigue. These symptoms are possibly thought of as an expected consequence of treatment or may require a longer period of time before the symptom is resolved once action is taken.

Patients who attempted to relieve symptoms either generated relief themselves or sought the aid of health care professionals. Health care providers were approached most often for pain, nausea and vomiting, sore mouth, trouble sleeping, burning on urination, fever, and swelling. Most patients attempted to relieve dry mouth, poor appetite, weight loss, weight gain, fatigue, and shortness of breath on their own.

Summary and Implications

The survey data presented here confirm the diverse literature reviewed with regard to the relationship between cancer patients' disease state and the likelihood that they will require assistance in meeting their daily living and special administrative needs. Generally, among patients undergoing active chemotherapy, those receiving adjuvant and curative treatment were less likely to experience the host of functional problems for which they require assistance than those receiving palliative therapy. Nonetheless, even among the group of higher need individuals, only a small minority were experiencing functional deficits that inhibited their performance of basic physical activities such as mobility and bathing.

Most patients requiring assistance needed help in performing the 'instrumental' activities of daily living, such as shopping, cooking, and getting to places including their medical appointments. Assistance with administrative functions such as completing insurance claim forms was more common among the sicker patients, suggesting that as the disease progresses, patients are more likely to be deluged with administrative tasks at a point when they are less able to cope with increasing disability. Expressed need for legal, financial, and treatment-related information and advice was less prevalent than requests for assistance with form completion, suggesting perhaps that patients are able to recognize and respond to the more concrete tasks and are less able to recognize longer range issues such as financial planning around the disease (if they exist).

Until relatively recently, the literature about the needs of patients and their families has generally emphasized the psychological and emotional dimensions. Patients' fears about their prognosis, depression, and sense of powerlessness have been examined and even considered as a determinant of survival [40–44]. Nonetheless, the interaction between physical (and consequently functional) decline associated with both disease progression or treatment and the patient's emotional condition has not been adequately explored, particularly in relation to the manner in which the patient might present to the treating physician. Physical decline and the inability to meet one's daily needs (or the fear of not being able to do so) has a powerful effect on patients' mood state. Mor [22] examined the relationship between physical functioning and depression in three samples of cancer patients: newly diagnosed, active chemotherapy, and terminal. In all samples the correlation was strong with depressed mood increasing as functioning declined. This relationship remained strong even after controlling for the severity of a patient's physical symptoms such as pain, nausea, and shortness of breath.

The most common type of interaction psychiatrists have with cancer patients is through consultation liaison to investigate issues ranging from threats of suicide to cognitive dysfunction associated with metastases to the brain. The literature to date has provided little guidance about the effect that the burden of coping with multiple concrete problems has on patients' emotional condition and capacity to adapt successfully to life-threatening illness. Prolonged feelings of physical exhaustion associated with trying to perform all daily activities independently could make patients more susceptible to depression, particularly when they finally must seek assistance. Additionally, the inability to have needs met places considerable strain on the patient and the family helping network that is generally involved.

In an earlier study, considerable evidence emerged for the appearance of emotional and interpersonal distress in response to the concrete burden of the cancer experience [19]. A majority of family caregivers reported mood disturbance in the form of negative feelings. Almost half experienced an increase in disagreements with other family members. This overlay of emotional dysfunction in the context of concrete need presents a challenge for psychiatric assessment. When patients and families are uninformed with regard to possible resources, their ability to articulate their needs to a care provider will be substantially limited. It is very likely that they would approach a clinician with complaints of distress rather than a request for specific services. Given the fact that the majority of subjects in the study described in this chapter, who were not yet involved with service agencies, could not identify formal sources of assistance, a crisis-oriented approach is likely to be the norm. Conversely, those patients and families with significant psychiatric disturbance may be more impaired in negotiating with social and concrete service agencies and may become dysfunctional in response to the burden of combined complex problems. A multidisciplinary approach that covers the social aspects of the world confronting the patient must be adopted in order to sort out the interplay between concrete needs and psychiatric symptoms. The medical model cannot fully account for the variety of ways in which patients present with symptoms of distress or the forms of intervention necessary to alleviate them.

Patients with an excess of concrete needs, and particularly those not receiving sufficient assistance, may present themselves as being emotionally distraught and with psychiatric symptoms such as anxiety and depression. Before approaching the patient's condition with medications to quell the symptoms, it may be more important to investigate the extent to which problems, fears, and frustrations with the treatment system or concerns about finances are contributing to the picture. At least some such concrete needs can be met relatively simply by providing patients with home health or transportation services. Our data suggest that few patients are aware of the availability of such services and do not have clear strategies as to how they might alleviate their problems. Before altering patients' experiences of their symptoms, it may be wise to educate them as to the availability of services and encourage and guide them to secure the assistance they need.

References

1 Yancik, R.: Frame of reference: old age as the context for the prevention and treatment of cancer; in Perspectives on prevention and treatment of cancer in the elderly (Raven Press, New York 1983).
2 Cairns, J.: Aging and the natural history of cancer; in Perspectives on prevention and treatment of cancer in the elderly (Raven Press, New York 1983).
3 Janerich, D.T.: Forecasting cancer trends to optimize control strategies. J. natn. Cancer Inst. *72:* 1317–1321 (1984).
4 Feldman, A.R.; Kessler, L.; Myers, M.H.; Naughton, M.D.: The prevalence of cancer. New Engl. J. Med. *315:* 1394–1397 (1986).
5 Schottenfeld, D.: Fundamental issues in cancer screening in colorectal cancer; in Colorectal cancer: prevention, epidemiology and screening (Raven Press, New York 1980).
6 Chodak, G.W.; Schoenberg, H.W.: Early detection of prostate cancer by routine screening. J. Am. med. Ass. *252:* 3261–3264 (1984).
7 Kronborg, O.: Mass screening for colorectal cancer. Scand. J. Gastroent. *19:* 1–5 (1984).
8 Ermann, D.; Gabel, J.: Emergency centers, and surgery centers. Med. Care *23:* 401–420 (1984).
9 Mor, V.; Laliberte, L.; Hiris, J.; Cryan, C.; Schwartz, R.; Masterson-Allen, S.: The impact of an adult day hospital on the lives of cancer patients and families and on health care costs. In connection with a Robert Wood Johnson Foundation contract to Memorial Sloan-Kettering Cancer Center (October 1986).
10 Herz, M.I.; Endicott, J.; Spitzer, R.L.; Mesnikoff, A.: Day versus inpatient hospitalization: a controlled study. Am. J. Psych. *127:* 1371–1382 (1971).
11 Herz, M.I.: Research overview in day treatment. Int. J. part. Hospital. *1:* 33–44 (1982).
12 Isler, C.: Emerging in cancer care: the regional ambulatory center. RN Mag. (1977).

13 Mason, J.C.; Louks, J.L.; Burmer, G.C.; Scher, M.: The efficacy of partial hospitalization: a review of recent literature. Int. J. part. Hospital. *1:* 251–269 (1982).
14 Moscowitz, I.S.: The effectiveness of day hospital treatment: a review. J. Community Psychol. *8:* 155–164 (1980).
15 Nirenberg, A.; Rosen, G.: The day hospital: ambulatory care. Am. J. Nurs. *79:* 500–504 (1979).
16 Ratkowski, E.; Liebermann, R.; Hochman, A.: Day care for cancer patients. J. Am. med. Ass. *230:* 430–431 (1974).
17 Walker, G.M.; Foster, R.S.; McKegney, C.T.; McKegney, F.T.: Breast biopsy: a comparison of outpatient and inpatient experiences. Archs Surg. *113:* 942–946 (1978).
18 Wilkes, E.; Crowther, A.G.O.; Greaves, E.W.K.H.J.: A different kind of day hospital — for patients with preterminal cancer and chronic disease. Br. med. J. *ii:* 1053–1056 (1978).
19 Mor, V.; Guadagnoli, E.; Wool, M.: An examination of the concrete service needs of advanced cancer patients. J. psychosoc. Oncol. *5:* 1–17 (1987).
20 Houts, P.; Yasko, J.; Kahn, S.; Schelzel, G.; Maroni, K.: Unmet psychological, social and economic needs of persons with cancer in Pennsylvania. Cancer *58:* 2355–2361 (1986).
21 Ganz, P.A.; Schag, C.C.; Heinrich, R.L.: The psychosocial impact of cancer on the elderly: a comparison with younger patients. J. Am. Geriat. Soc. *33:* 429–435 (1985).
22 Mor, V.: Cancer patients' quality of life over the disease course: lessons from the real world. J. chron. Dis. *40:* 535–544 (1987).
23 Somers, A.R.: The changing demand for health services: a historical perspective and some thoughts for the future. Inquiry *23:* 395–402 (1986).
24 Cassileth, B.R.; Lusk, E.J.; Strouse, T.B.; Miller, D.S.; Brown, L.L.; Cross, P.A.: A psychological analysis of cancer patients and their next-of-kin. Cancer *55:* 72–76 (1985).
25 Weisman, A.D.; Worden, J.W.; Sobel, H.J.: Psychosocial screening and intervention with cancer patients. Final report of the Omega Project, NCI Grant No. CA-19797 (Boston 1980).
26 Weisman, A.D.: A model for psychosocial phasing in cancer. Gen. Hosp. Psychiat. *1:* 187–195 (1979).
27 Heinrich, R.L.; Schag, C.C.; Ganz, P.A.: Living with cancer: the cancer inventory of problem situations. J. clin. Psychol. *40:* 972–980 (1984).
28 Gold, M.: Life support: families speak about hospital, hospice, and home care for the fatally ill (Institute for Consumer Policy Research, Consumers Union Foundation, Mount Vernon 1983).
29 Schomberg, F.L.; Pascasio, A.; Lippincott, R.C.; Nicholas, J.J.: Demonstration of cancer rehabilitation facilities and/or departments; in Multidisciplinary functional approach for rehabilitation of patients with cancer. Prepared under contract with the National Cancer Institute (Nol-CN-55-298) (School of Health Related Professions, University of Pittsburgh, Pittsburgh 1978).
30 Greer, D.S.; Mor, V.; Morris, J.N.; Sherwood, S.; Kidder, D.; Birnbaum, H.: An alternative in terminal care: results of the National Hospice Study. J. chron. Dis. *39:* 9–26 (1986).
31 Mor, V.; Masterson-Allen, S.: Hospice care systems: structure, process, costs, and outcome (Springer, New York 1987).

32 Pfeiffer, E.: Multidimensional functional assessment: the OARS methodology (Center for the Study of Aging and Human Development, Duke University, Durham 1975).
33 Little, V.C.: Assessing the needs of the elderly: state of the art. Int. J. Aging hum. Dev. *11:* 65–76 (1980).
34 Stengle, W.A.; Eckert, D.: Colorectal cancer patients' rehabilitation and continuing care needs: a preliminary assessment of services provided by a voluntary cancer agency; in Progress in cancer control, part IV, pp. 433–442 (Liss, New York 1983).
35 Selby, P.J.; Chapman, J.A.; Etazadi-Amoli, J.; Dalley, D.; Boyd, N.F.: The development of a method for assessing the quality of life of cancer patients. Br. J. Cancer *50:* 13–22 (1984).
36 Lehmann, J.F.; DeLisa, J.A.; Warren, C.G.; deLateur, B.J.; Bryant, P.L.S.; Nicholson, C.G.: Cancer rehabilitation: assessment of need, development, and evaluation of a model of care. Archs phys. Med. Rehabil. *59:* 410–419 (1978).
37 Craig, T.J.; Comstock, G.W.; Geiser, P.B.: Quality of survival in breast cancer: care-control comparison. Cancer *33:* 1451–1457 (1974).
38 Feldman, J.G.; Gardner, B.; Carter, A.C.; Alfonso, A.; Orces, H.: Relationship of race to functional status among breast cancer patients after curative surgery. J. surg. Oncol. *11:* 333–339 (1979).
39 Spector, W.D.; Katz, S.; Murphy, J.B.; Fulton, J.P.: The hierarchical relationship between activities of daily living and instrumental activities of daily living. J. chron. Dis. *40:* 481–489 (1987).
40 Fox, B.H.: Current theory of psychogenic effects on cancer incidence and prognosis. J. psychosoc. Oncol. *1:* 17–31 (1983).
41 Derogatis, L.R.; Abeloff, M.D.; Melisaratos, N.: Psychosocial coping mechanisms and survival time in metastatic breast cancer. J. Am. med. Ass. *242:* 1504–1508 (1979).
42 Greer, H.S.; Morris, T.; Pettingale, K.W.: Psychological response to breast cancer: effect on outcome. Lancet *ii:* 785–787 (1979).
43 Pettingale, K.W.; Morris, T.; Greer, S.; Haybittle, J.L.: Mental attitudes to cancer: an additional prognostic factor. Lancet *i:* 750 (1985).
44 Cassileth, B.R.; Lusk, E.J.; Miller, D.S.; Brown, L.L.; Miller, C.: Psychosocial correlates of survival in advanced malignant disease? New Engl. J. Med. *312:* 1551–1555 (1985).
45 American Cancer Society: Report on the social, economic and psychological needs of cancer patients in California (Greenleigh Associates, San Francisco 1979).
46 Grobe, M.E.; Ahmann, D.L.; Ilstrup, D.M.: Needs assessment for advanced cancer patients and their families. Oncol. Nurs. Forum. *9:* 26–30 (1982).
47 Houts, P.S.: Psychological, social and economic needs of persons with cancer in Pennsylvania. Interim report (Pennsylvania State University College of Medicine, Hershey 1985).

Vincent Mor, PhD, Center for Health Care Research, Brown University,
Box G, Providence, RI 02912 (USA)

Adv. psychosom. Med., vol. 18, pp. 119–134 (Karger, Basel 1988)

The Hospice Model of Care for the Terminally Ill[1]

Vincent Mor, Susan Masterson-Allen

Brown University, Center for Health Care Research, Providence, R.I., USA

Background: The Evolution of Hospice

Advances in medical technology and public health practices have led to a dramatic demographic shift in American society in the last century. Better medical care and miracle vaccines resulted in a decline in infant mortality and an arrest of infectious diseases which once claimed the lives of the young and the very young [Halper, 1979; Ryder and Ross, 1977]. Declines in both fertility and mortality, combined with an increase in longevity, have shifted the age distribution of the population so that the proportion of people over the age of 65 jumped from 4% in 1900 to approximately 12% today [Fox, 1981]. The fastest growing segment of the population is the 85-and-over age group. By the end of the century, numbers in this group will have doubled.

While medical research has succeeded in controlling many of the communicable diseases, efforts to cure chronic, degenerative diseases or, as in the case of cancer, to even comprehend the biological mechanisms that trigger the disease, have been less successful. Chronic, long-term diseases are the primary cause of death in the USA today. An estimated 965,000 people will be newly diagnosed with cancer in 1987, and approximately 483,000 deaths will occur as a result of the disease [ACS, 1987]. As it is the elderly who are most at risk for contracting these diseases, death has become a phenomenon of the aged. Some 80% of people dying in the USA today are over the age of 65 [Halper, 1979; Fisher et al., 1983].

Over the past decade, the role of the modern hospital in serving the chronically and terminally ill has been questioned [Krant, 1978; Lack, 1978;

[1] This work was supported in part by DHHS/HCFA Grant No. 99-P-97793 and grants from the Robert Wood Johnson Foundation and the John A. Hartford Foundation.

Saunders, 1978]. The technologically oriented health care system which emphasizes diagnosis, treatment, and cure is felt to be irrelevant when cure is no longer a possibility [Kastenbaum, 1969].

Hospice emerged in the UK in the late 1960s and in the USA in the early 1970s. It arose out of a dissatisfaction with modern medicine's approach to caring for the terminal patient, society's increased willingness to talk about death and dying, and a sober realization of the rising cost of health care. In the USA, hospice as a concept inspired a groundswell of support that became a social movement [Holden, 1980]. Groups of individuals in communities across the country formed to discuss strategies to alter the existing approach to treating the terminally ill. Some groups chose to create 'alternative' systems for meeting patients' needs, while others sought to catalyze the existing health care system to become more sensitive to the needs of the dying patient.

Hospice, as an organizational delivery system, made its appearance in the USA in 1974 with the opening of Hospice, Inc. in New Haven, Connecticut. Estimates from the Joint Commission on Accreditation of Hospitals (JCAH) and the National Hospice Organization suggest that there are about 1,694 hospices across the country serving over 100,000 patients [NHO, 1985b]. More a philosophy of care than an institutional entity, hospice espouses palliative rather than curative care, the patient and family as the unit of care, and the administration of care by an interdisciplinary team whose members are geared toward meeting the unique needs of terminally ill patients and their families.

Support for hospice from most sectors of American society was so strong that its proponents were able to successfully introduce Congressional legislation in support of hospice care. At a time when Congress and the Administration were interested in cutting programs and costs, hospice was introduced as a new benefit under Medicare. This was done as a part of the Tax Equity and Fiscal Responsibility Act (TEFRA) in 1982. A mere 8 years after the founding of the first American hospice, it became a Medicare-covered service.

The prominent features of the hospice legislation and regulation included the following stipulations [Greer and Mor, 1985]: (1) A patient eligibility requirement of a physician-certified prognosis of 6 months or less. (2) A limitation of $6,500 reimbursement per patient times the number of patients served by a particular hospice (this has subsequently been increased). (3) A limitation of 210 days of coverage per patient, with no more than 20% of this time spent in an inpatient setting. (4) Mandatory availability in all hospices of both home nursing services and hospice inpatient care. (5) A provision that the Hospice Interdisciplinary Team must maintain financial and clinical control of all patient care in both home and inpatient settings. (6) Mandatory provision by all hospices of ministerial, bereavement, and volunteer services, although these services are not directly reimbursable.

A 'sunset clause', stipulating that the law would expire without additional Congressional action, was appended to the legislation as a safeguard against possible unanticipated consequences of reimbursing a new health care system. This clause required a reassessment of the feasibility of reimbursing hospice services within 3 years from the date the benefit went into effect (October 1, 1983). However, the Sunset provision was repealed in 1986, thus conferring Federal sanction on hospice as a legitimate component of the health care system.

In addition to the legislative legitimation granted hospice, the nation's largest private health care insurer, Blue Cross and Blue Shield Association, added hospice coverage to its Federal employees and retirees plan. 'It (the hospice benefit) will emphasize care at home and cover an extensive range of home care services, although there will be a $3,000 maximum. Five days of hospice inpatient care will be covered. There will be no payment for bereavement services. Local plans will approve hospice programs for participation in this benefit' [NHO, 1985a]. Other evidence of broad support for the concept came from a survey of 1,115 employers conducted by a benefits consulting firm which revealed that more than 40% of employers responding included hospice care as a benefit in their group plans. As of 1985, legislatures in seven states have passed laws requiring that insurance plans offer a hospice benefit [Moga, 1985; NHO, 1986]. Although coverage varies widely and in some cases is insufficient, the trend is indicative of hospice's acceptance by third-party payers.

There is general agreement among observers of the hospice movement that the 1982 legislation enabling a hospice benefit under Medicare contributed to the transformation of hospice from innovation to medical mainstream [Tehan, 1985; Abel, 1986; Paradis and Cummings, 1986]. The tone of published commentary is typically one of mild disappointment and resignation to the inevitable dilution of the hospice philosophy as focus shifts to organizational survival within a competitive system.

Although the fervor of the hospice movement has diminished, the majority of hospice advocates are encouraged by the national recognition of the validity of hospice's approach to care for the terminally ill. 'Success has brought uniformity and fiscal constraints, but the commitment to "low-tech, high-touch" care has not changed' [Tehan, 1985].

The following pages describe the hospice system of care for the terminally ill in the USA today. Recognizing that individual aspects of hospice organizations vary, we have attempted to characterize hospice staff, organizational arrangements, patients, and services provided that are typical yet convey the alternative nature of the hospice delivery system. Additionally, we review available knowledge on the cost effectiveness of hospice and its success in achieving positive quality of life outcomes. Much of the information presented here emanates from the two most comprehensive hospice evaluation projects conducted to date, a randomized clinical trial of patients admitted to a hospice unit in a Veterans Administration Hospital [Kane et al., 1984] and the National Hospice Study (NHS), a nonrandomized, multisite trial of the cost effectiveness of different models of hospice care [Greer et al., 1986].

Hospice Organizational Structure

Three types of hospice organizational structures have evolved, each with numerous variations. They are: (1) hospices affiliated with hospitals, with or without a home care component; (2) hospices affiliated with preexisting home health agencies, without their own inpatient unit, and (3) hospices that emerged as organizations exclusively serving terminal patients, with or without a special inpatient unit. The variations that exist include nursing homes, replacing the hospital as the parent provider, and quasi-independent coordinating groups that create hospice programs from the collaborative efforts of existing agencies.

One effect of TEFRA on hospice is evident when we compare the organizational structure of hospices which have sought Medicare certification with that of all known operational hospices. Home health affiliated hospices, which represent only 18% of all known hospices, constitute 44% of the certified hospices. Freestanding hospices are 25% of all certified hospices and yet make up 40% of the entire population of hospices. The proportion of hospital-based, certified hospices is 21%, an underrepresentation of nearly 10%. Finally, although skilled nursing facilities (SNF) comprise only 1% of the total population of hospices, they make up 4% of certified hospices. As SNF represent a proprietary interest in hospice care, their representation can be expected to increase in the future.

From the outset, the hospice movement has been dominated by the nonprofit voluntary sector. The first hospices were run by community groups and health care providers who had a strong sense of community mission. Perhaps since hospice services were not reimbursable until recently, proprietary interests have stayed out of the 'hospice market'. However, as additional experience under the Medicare benefit is accrued and other insurers now offer hospice as a reimbursable benefit, we may expect to see the entry of proprietary hospice providers into the system.

Hospice leadership structure appears to be related to the organizational origins of hospices. Those started by community groups tend to have community boards of people from diverse backgrounds. In contrast, hospices developed by health care professionals are likely to be led by representatives from the health professions.

Both the TEFRA legislation and guidelines specified by the JCAH state that a hospice must be able to provide the full range of patient services if it is to maintain clinical control over care. The lack of start-up monies for service development and integration, however, significantly affects the range of services hospices provide. Most hospices directly provide some services and contract for the provision of others. Some organizations call themselves hospices but do not offer the full range of hospice services. They often provide only psychosocial services.

Nonetheless, most hospice programs described in the literature provide a set of services that conforms with the National Hospice Organization's model of a hospice program [NHO, 1979]. Paradis [1984] reports in her survey of over 40 hospice programs in Michigan that the majority provide or arrange for the following services: (1) basic skilled nursing; (2) companionship; (3) psychological counseling; (4) personal care; (5) symptom control; (6) social work; (7) bereavement counseling; (8) housekeeping; (9) transportation and errands; (10) meal preparation, and (11) education about hospice.

Hospice Patients

The hospice movement has grown so fast in the last decade that most major population centers have at least one hospice. A survey conducted by the National Hospice Organization estimates that in 1984 over 100,000 patients were served by hospices throughout the USA [NHO, 1985b]. The most reliable way of describing the characteristics of hospice patients is from the hospice research literature. Fourteen reports were identified which presented hospice patient characteristics [Mor and Masterson-Allen, 1987]. A total of 15,119 patients are represented by these studies, 13,374 of whom were served by National Hospice Study sites. In the paragraphs below, we attempt to draw generalizations about patients of hospice care.

Just over one half of hospice patients are female, and the large majority are white (approximately 90% across studies). Nonwhites and hispanics appear to be underrepresented in hospice use. The National Hospice Study found the percentage of nonwhites was less than 8% and the percentage of hispanics was about 4%. In contrast, their representation in cancer deaths is in proportion to their representation in the general population.

Across all studies, the average age appears to be in the mid to upper sixties, a 'young-old' clientele. It is interesting to note the marked contrast between the age distribution of hospice patients and that of nursing home patients. The large majority of nursing home residents are over the age of 75, with approximately one third being over 85.

A uniform characteristic of hospice patients across studies is that they have a primary care person to assist with their care. Data from the literature indicate that the primary care person is the patient's spouse over 50% of the time. In another 18–33% of cases, the patient's child fills the caretaking role. It is evident that the nature of the hospice intervention requires a strong informal support system, particularly for home care hospice patients.

The length of hospice stay is a crucial indicator of the composition of patients admitted; it often correlates closely with the intensity of the resources required on a daily basis. Length of stay of hospice patients is strongly related to their functional status and nursing care needs at the time of admission [Mor and Hiris, 1983]. The NHS showed that 51% of all hospital-based hospice patients had a length of stay under 22 days, compared with 38% of home care patients. This suggests that patients who are closer to death may have more severe care requirements likely to require inpatient care. In general, the median length of stay across the various studies examined is between 30 and 45 days.

The results of studies on hospice patient mix show that most (over 90%) patients who choose hospice have cancer as their diagnosis. It appears that about 20% of hospice patients have respiratory problems which require oxygen (this is only slightly less than the average percentage of hospice patients with lung cancer).

Caretakers of the Terminally Ill

Care for the terminally ill patient requires a comprehensive, coordinated approach that deals with the patient's medical, social, psychological, and spiritual needs over a period of time. Hospice care addresses these needs through the hospice interdisciplinary team (HIT). Among the professionals reported in the literature as partaking in the hospice team are physicians, nurses, psychologists, social workers, dieticians, physical/occupational therapists, pharmacists, and volunteers [Winstead et al., 1980; JCAH, 1984]. The team constructs a care plan to meet all the patient's needs and also serves to provide mutual support to staff in resolving problems, coping with stress, and offering medical assistance. It is largely this interdisciplinary approach that makes the hospice intervention unique.

Hospice is primarily a nursing intervention. In no area of health care is nursing professionalism as obvious as in hospice care, in which good nursing care, not physician's cure, is the ultimate objective. Although not as prominent as in an acute care setting, the physician is, nevertheless, an important member of the hospice team. JCAH standards require the attending physician's signature on the team care plan to indicate knowledge and approval of services to be provided [JCAH, 1984]. Both Medicare and JCAH require hospices to have a medical director.

In addition to nurses and physicians, the National Hospice Study found that 13.7% of hospice staff were other direct care staff such as social workers, bereavement counselors, and occupational, physical, and nutritional therapists. Administrators (who might also have been clinically involved in the program) and clerical workers comprised another 20% of hospice staff.

The volunteer is central to both hospice philosophy and operation. In fact, the availability of volunteer services is mandatory under TEFRA regulations for Medicare eligibility. Volunteers are used to supplement the caregiving capacity of the hospice as well as to assist in the role of administrative and community liaison. The role of volunteers in hospice can best be described as supportive — to patients, their families, and paid staff [Mantell and Ell, 1985; Mor and Laliberte, 1983].

The Process of Hospice Care

The hospice movement has unquestionably altered the manner in which care for the terminally ill patient is conceptualized and delivered. Hospice standards, emphasizing a palliative approach to care, were developed early in the course of the movement's development by proponents who were committed to establishing a uniform philosophy and process of care. Three major trends which emerge in the literature are: (1) a focus on pain and symptom control; (2) concern with clinical control in relation to continuity of care, and (3) emphasis on psychosocial issues pertaining to the care of terminally ill patients and their families.

Pain and Symptom Control. Controlling patients' pain and symptoms is one of the primary goals of hospice care. Those in the vanguard of the hospice movement felt that their central contribution was to the technology of pain and symptom control. Baines [1984] outlines a series of principles of pain control used at St. Christopher's Hospice in England. These embody the basic approach to pain control in both British and American hospices today: (1) cancer pain is continuous and needs prevention; (2) analgesic dose should be the lowest compatible with pain control; (3) titrate the dose until the patient is pain-free; (4) administer doses on a regular, preventive schedule; (5) oral medication is preferable; (6) dependence is not an issue; (7) tolerance is only a minor problem and is usually self-limiting; (8) continual reassessment and monitoring is needed for old and new pains; (9) adjuvant therapy using laxatives and other agents to prevent nausea and constipation is usually necessary.

Clinical Control of Care. According to both the hospice legislation and the philosophy of the hospice movement, the entire patient care plan should be infused with hospice principles. To assure continuity of care, control of the clinical course of care is essential. Clinical control is also important because of Medicare-certified hospices' fiscal liability for all care received by their patients. Under the TEFRA legislation, once a patient becomes a hospice patient, the hospice serves as a type of health maintenance organization (HMO). This means that if the patient at home is admitted to a hospital without the written authorization of the hospice, the costs incurred may be the responsibility of the patient: like an HMO, all care must be preauthorized. Consequently, for both clinical and fiscal purposes, it is critical that the hospice establish systems to ensure both continuity and control of patient care.

The major area of 'gate-keeping' for the hospice is that of inpatient admissions. Obviously, this process is facilitated when the inpatient unit is part of the hospice. According to the JCAH survey of hospice programs

[1984], over 100 of 345 respondents provided no inpatient care. All of these were community-based, home care hospices. The hospice interdisciplinary team has no control over the pattern of care when patients are admitted to a hospital inpatient setting. Legal authority to prescribe care is vested in the patient's physician and, by extension, the house staff. Therefore, the hospice team may find it impossible to impose their approved plan of care in that situation.

Control over the provision of home care services is equally important. In spite of the Medicare requirement that home nursing be substantially provided by hospice staff, a large proportion of hospices contract for home care services. In many cases, this is to supplement care provided by their own staff. Hospital-based and freestanding hospices are much more likely to contract for home care services than are home health agency-based hospices. A partial solution to the problem of maintaining clinical control is case management, the coordination of patient care across settings.

Patient Psychological Care and Counseling. Over the past two decades, a considerable literature has developed regarding approaches to assist the terminally ill through the psychological process of dying [Kastenbaum and Aisenburg, 1972; Kübler-Ross, 1969]. In particular, patients' denial of their illness has been studied by numerous investigators and clinicians [Mount, 1980; Weisman, 1979]. Terminal cancer patients entering hospice do not always acknowledge their disease and prognosis, despite the fact that they may have signed informed consent documents on entry to the program. In the National Hospice Study, as many as 15% of terminal cancer hospice patients already receiving services did not acknowledge their diagnosis. Older patients, those not admitted to freestanding hospice settings, and those diagnosed relatively recently were more likely not to acknowledge the diagnosis of cancer. The implications for hospice staff are obvious: special attention must be paid to discussion of the patient's prognosis.

Depression is a common symptom in the terminal population [Goldberg, 1981; Derogatis et al., 1983]. However, it is often difficult to determine if depressive symptoms such as impaired sleep or appetite are attributed to the physical consequences of the illness or to a psychological adjustment reaction. Effective intervention depends on the correct identification of etiology. A comprehensive approach to the depressed cancer patient involves addressing physical, psychological, social, and existential dimensions.

Family Bereavement Counseling. Relief of the psychological and physical distress associated with bereavement has become a major objective of the hospice movement in the USA. Even before the emergence of the hospice movement, a large body of literature had begun to emerge describing the psychological and physiological adjustment processes experienced by the bereaved [Osterweis et al., 1984].

Bereavement programs have always been a part of hospice for at least two reasons: the interpretation of the patient and family as a single unit of care, and the contemporaneous development of a focus upon the needs of the terminally ill and the needs of the bereaved. The techniques employed by hospices in their bereavement programs range from group counseling, to support groups sponsored rather than operated by the hospice, to individual psychotherapy, to periodic social events for survivors with a common experience of loss.

Quality of Life Outcomes

The benefits claimed by the hospice movement are both global and specific [Saunders, 1981]. They pertain to both the patient and the family [NHO, 1979] and should be observable as patients proceed through the normal stages of disease progression and deterioration [Greer et al., 1983]. The outcomes most relevant to hospice are: pain and symptom control, site of death, satisfaction with care received, patient and family psychosocial outcomes, and family bereavement outcomes. Based upon available evaluation studies, the success of hospice in achieving positive outcomes in these areas is described below.

Pain and Symptom Control. Available research suggests that the prevalence of pain in the terminally ill is between 30 and 60%. Evaluation studies demonstrate that hospice does not result in patients experiencing more pain. Indeed, some comparison studies report that hospice may achieve small but significant positive differences in achieving pain control [Greer et al., 1986; Morris et al., 1986]. These differences, however, seem to be observable only when the base rates of pain in the study population are relatively high and when informants comment upon the patient's condition.

While hospice philosophy is generally associated with pain control, the focus on palliation suggests that the prevalence and severity of symptoms such as dyspnea, nausea, vomiting, and other gastrointestinal symptoms, as

well as indicators of cognitive functioning, may be lower in hospice. Kane et al. [1984, 1985a] found no significant difference between hospice and nonhospice patients on the number and severity of symptoms reported. While the NHS found a statistically significant difference in the number of different symptoms reported by patients' families (to the benefit of hospital-based hospices), this effect was not isolated to any given symptom such as nausea or dyspnea [Greer et al., 1986; Reuben and Mor, 1986].

Site of Death. Reports from the literature reveal that between 30 and 72% of patients served in hospice-type programs which emphasize home care die at home. Between 20 and 30% of patients served in hospices with inpatient units die at home. In contrast, and consistent with the national data, between 15 and 20% of cancer patients served by conventional oncological systems die at home [Mor and Hiris, 1983]. Thus, it appears that hospice facilitates home death for those patients and families who desire it. There are, however, differences in the likelihood of home death between the two models of hospice care. Although there are differences in the mix of patients served in the two settings [Mor et al., 1985; Mor and Hiris, 1983], the magnitude of the difference in home death rates is not likely to be explained by patient characteristics alone. Rather, the systems and philosophies of care appear to differ. Since home death is not necessarily a universal 'good', it is reasonable that the hospice movement allows for choice.

Satisfaction with Care. In spite of the differences in methods and the vast diversity of measures used across studies, it appears that patients served in hospices are more satisfied with the care they receive than are nonhospice patients. There is some indication, however, that this positive effect may be associated particularly with the inpatient variety of hospice.

The NHS found that although home care patients' family members were satisfied, they were not significantly more satisfied than were nonhospice patients' families. The one area in which both home care and hospital-based families were more satisfied than were nonhospice patients' families was in site of death [Greer et al., 1986].

Patient Psychosocial Outcomes. Neither the NHS nor the VA Hospital hospice evaluation found differences between hospice and comparison patients with regard to psychosocial outcomes. Kane et al. [1985b] found no differences in either depression or anxiety (as measured by standardized scales) between hospice and control terminal cancer patients. The National

Hospice Study [Greer et al., 1986] found similar results using a rating of emotional state as perceived by the patients' caretaker. The prevalence of depression and serious anxiety and mood disturbance were fairly low in all of these studies.

If we can generalize from the studies conducted to date, it would appear that the hospice 'aura' and philosophy do not have the indirect effect on patients' psychological state that has been supposed. On the other hand, the measures used by existing studies may not have been sufficiently sensitive or specific to detect the effect hospice does have on patients' psychosocial status.

Bereavement Outcomes. The NHS found no significant differences between hospice and nonhospice primary care persons in terms of concrete indicators of secondary morbidity as measured by hospitalization, physician visits, increased alcohol use, use of medications for anxiety, or thoughts of suicide in the 4 months following the death of the patient. There were significant differences between home care and hospital-based hospice primary care persons in terms of the proportion of respondents reporting depression and severe grief reaction (hospital-based family members reported them less often); however, no statistically significant differences were observed between either hospice group and conventional care survivors.

Kane et al. [1986] studied the impact of bereavement on a sample of 56 'significant others' associated with hospice patients and 40 'significant others' of control patients. Results indicate a decrease in depression and anxiety over time for both groups. However, there was no significant difference between groups on either measure. Kane's study was consistent with the NHS in not finding differences in indicators of secondary morbidity even one year after the death of the patient. These results must be a source of great disappointment to hospice proponents, since psychosocial care for the family and patient is central to the hospice philosophy.

The Cost-Effectiveness of Hospice Care

Studies which have investigated the cost of providing hospice care reveal substantial variation, particularly by whether the hospice has inpatient beds and the length of stay of patients served in the hospice [Mor and Kidder, 1985; Birnbaum and Kidder, 1984; Kane et al., 1984]. At present, we have insufficient information to know whether the variation in hospice costs is broader than cost variations in other sectors of the health care industry. What is likely, however, is that the cost of hospice services will change as the industry grows and as more hospices become certified and enter the environment of prospective payment.

For hospice to result in cost savings, patients' costs and patterns of service use must differ from those in general terminal cancer patient populations. Terminal cancer patients' costs increase rapidly as death approaches, particularly hospital utilization costs [Lubitz et al., 1981; Spector and Mor, 1984; Mor and Kidder, 1985]. A potential outcome of hospice is that patients may begin receiving services earlier in their terminal course than they would if they were not in hospice. For hospice to be cost-effective, these additional early costs cannot exceed the savings that are generated by lower inpatient utilization in the last months of life.

The available literature strongly suggests that the home care hospice model achieves the goal of substituting home care for inpatient care [Mor and Kidder, 1985; Greer et al., 1986; Brooks and Smyth-Staruch, 1984]. The net result is savings that are between 10 and 20% of total health care costs in the last year of life. The hospital-based hospice model appears to add the home care services early in the terminal phase, as does the home care model, but there is more inpatient care in the final month of life among hospital-based hospice patients, nearly as much as there is among nonhospice patients. The only major cost advantage of hospital-based hospices appears to be relatively less intensive use of ancillary services such as diagnostic tests and procedures [Mor and Kidder, 1985].

For hospice to be less costly than conventional care, the family must bear some burden of care in the home. Evidence from the National Hospice Study reveals that families of hospice patients do assume the emotional and physical burden of many hours of direct care daily. In addition, these families incur substantial economic losses entailed in absence from the labor force [Muurinen, 1986]. These factors must be taken into consideration as the health care policies which advocate dehospitalization are debated.

Conclusions

Hospice is both a philosophy and a system of care which serves an end-stage cancer patient population. It is characterized by a multiplicity of organizational arrangements, all of which provide palliative rather than curative care, with an emphasis on symptom control and psychosocial support. The patient and family are the unit of care. Hospice is primarily a nursing intervention, with individualized care plans developed by an interdisciplinary team of health care professionals. The nature of the hospice intervention requires that patients have strong family support systems.

Evaluation results indicate that the hospice model of care may have some small positive effect on symptom control. Hospice also appears to yield increased satisfaction with care when compared to nonhospice patients, particularly regarding where patients die. However, comparison studies conducted to date have not detected differences in patient and family psychosocial outcomes when comparing hospice and conventional care.

Hospice has not been found to increase the cost of terminal care and, when delivered by the home care model, results in substantial savings compared to the costs incurred by patients in the conventional care system. The cost of hospice care delivered by the hospital-based model does not appear to be substantially less than nonhospice care. In conclusion, since hospice costs no more and apparently has no negative effects, from a social policy perspective it is a viable alternative for those patients and families who prefer a palliative, nontechnological approach to terminal care.

References

Abel, E.K.: The hospice movement: institutionalizing innovation. Int. J. Hlth Serv. *16:* 71–85 (1986).

American Cancer Society: Cancer facts and figures — 1987 (Am. Cancer Society, New York 1987).

Baines, M.J.: Cancer pain. Post grad. med. J. *60:* 852–857 (1984).

Birnbaum, H.G.; Kidder, D.: What does hospice cost? Am. J. publ. Hlth *74:* 689–697 (1984).

Brooks, C.H.; Smyth-Staruch, K.: Hospice home care cost savings to third-party insurers. Med. Care *22:* 691–703 (1984).

Derogatis, L.R.; Morrow G.R.; Fetting, J.; Penman, D.; Piasetsky, S.; Schmale, A.M.; Henrichs, M.; Carnicke, C.L.M.: The prevalence of psychiatric disorder among cancer patients. J. Am. med. Ass. *249:* 751–757 (1983).

Fisher, R.H.; Nadon, G.W.; Shedletsky, R.: Management of the dying elderly patient. J. Am. Geriat. Soc. *31:* 563–564 (1983).

Fox, R.C.: The sting of death in American society. Soc. Serv. Rev. *55:* 42–59 (1981).

Goldberg, R.J.: Management of depression in the patient with advanced cancer. J. Am. med. Ass. *246:* 373–376 (1981).

Greer, D.S.; Mor, V.: How Medicare is altering the hospice movement. Hastings Cent. Rep. *15:* 5–10 (1985).

Greer, D.S.; Mor, V.; Morris, J.N.; Sherwood, S.; Kidder, D.; Birnbaum, H.: An alternative in terminal care: results of the National Hospice Study. J. chron. Dis. *39:* 9–26 (1986).

Greer, D.S.; Mor, V.; Sherwood, S.; Morris, J.N.; Birnbaum, H.: National Hospice Study analysis plan. J. chron. Dis. *36:* 737–780 (1983).

Halper, T.: On death, dying, and terminality: today, yesterday, and tomorrow. J. Hlth Polit. Policy Law *4:* 11–29 (1979).
Holden, C.: The hospice movement and its implications. Ann. Am. Acad. Pol. Soc. Sci. *1980:* 59–63.
Joint Commission on Accreditation of Hospitals: The hospice project; draft report of the W.K. Kellogg Foundation funded project (Joint Commission on Accreditation of Hospitals, Chicago 1984).
Kane, R.L.; Bernstein, L.; Wales, J.; Rothenberg, R.: Hospice effectiveness in controlling pain. J. Am. med. Ass. *253:* 2683–2686 (1985a).
Kane, R.L.; Klein, S.J.; Bernstein, L.; Rothenberg, R.: The role of hospice in reducing the impact of bereavement. J. chron. Dis. *39:* 735–742 (1986).
Kane, R.L.; Klein, S.J.; Bernstein, L.; Rothenberg, R.; Wales, J.: Hospice role in alleviating the emotional stress of terminal patients and their families. Med. Care *23:* 189–197 (1985b).
Kane, R.L.; Wales, J.; Bernstein, L.; Leibowitz, A.; Kaplan, S.: A randomised controlled trial of hospice care. Lancet *i:* 890–894 (1984).
Kastenbaum, R.: Psychological death; in Pearson, Death and dying: current issues in the treatment of the dying person, pp. 1–27 (Case Western University, Cleveland 1969).
Kastenbaum, R.; Aisenburg, R.: The psychology of death (Springer, New York 1972).
Krant, M.J.: Sounding board: the hospice movement. New Engl. J. Med. *299:* 546–549 (1978).
Kübler-Ross, E.: On death and dying (Macmillan, New York 1969).
Lack, S.A.: Hospice helps patients 'live until they die'. Hosp. Admin. Curr. *22:* 27–30 (1978).
Lubitz, J.; Gornick, M.; Prihoda, R.: Use and costs of Medicare services in the last year of life (DHHS/HCFA Office of Research, Demonstrations, and Statistics, Washington 1981).
Mantell, J.E.; Ell, K.O.: Hospice volunteer programs: a proposed agenda. Hospice J. *1:* 85–101 (1985).
Moga, D.N.: The hospice equation. Bus Hlth *2:* 7–11 (1985).
Mor, V.; Hiris, J.: Determinants of site of death among hospice cancer patients. J. Health soc. Behav. *24:* 375–385 (1983).
Mor, V.; Kidder, D.: Cost savings in hospice: final results of the National Hospice Study. Health Serv. Res. *20:* 407–422 (1985).
Mor, V.; Laliberte, L.: Roles ascribed to volunteers: an examination of different types of hospice organizations. Eval. Health Prof. *6:* 453–464 (1983).
Mor, V.; Masterson-Allen, S.: Hospice care systems: structure, process, costs, and outcome (Springer, New York 1987).
Mor, V.; Wachtel, T.J.; Kidder, D.: Patient predictors of hospice choice: hospital versus home care programs. Med. Care *23:* 1115–1119 (1985).
Morris, J.N.; Suissa, S.; Sherwood, S.; Wright, S.M.; Greer, D.: Last days: a study of the quality of life of terminally ill cancer patients. J. chron. Dis. *39:* 47–62 (1986).
Mount, B.M.: Psychological impact of urologic cancer. Cancer *45:* 1985–1992 (1980).
Muurinen, J.-M.: The economics of informal care: labor market effects in the National Hospice Study. Med. Care *24:* 1007–1017 (1986).
National Hospice Organization: Standards of a hospice program of care (National Hospice Organization, McLean 1979).

National Hospice Organization: Blue Cross adds national hospice benefit. NHO Hospice News *3:* 6 (1985a).
National Hospice Organization: Profile of hospices in US: NHO testifies before US health data committee. NHO Hospice News *3:* 3 (1985b).
National Hospice Organization: State hospice requirements. NHO Hospice News *4:* 3 (1986).
Osterweis, M.; Solomon, F.; Green, M.: Bereavement: reactions, consequences, and care (National Academy, Washington 1984).
Paradis, L.F.: Hospice program integration: an issue for policymakers. Death Educ. *8:* 383–398 (1984).
Paradis, L.F.; Cummings, S.B.: The evolution of hospice in America toward organizational homogeneity. J. Health soc. Behav. *27:* 370–386 (1986).
Reuben, D.B.; Mor, V.: Dyspnea in terminal cancer patients. Chest *89:* 234–236 (1986).
Ryder, C.F.; Ross, D.M.: Terminal care — issues and alternatives. Publ. Hlth Rep. *92:* 20–29 (1977).
Saunders, C.: Hospice care. Am. J. Med. *65:* 726–728 (1978).
Saunders, C.M.: The hospice: its meaning to patients and their physicians. Hosp. Pract. *16:* 93–108 (1981).
Spector, W.D.; Mor, V.: Utilization and charges for terminal cancer patients in Rhode Island. Inquiry *21:* 328–337 (1984).
Tehan, C.: Has success spoiled hospice? Hastings Cent. Rep. *15:* 10–13 (1985).
Weisman, A.D.: A model for psychosocial phasing in cancer. Gen. Hosp. Psychiat. *1:* 187–195 (1979).
Winstead, D.K.; Gilmore, M.; Dollar, R.; Miller, E.: Hospice consultation team: a new multidisciplinary model. Gen. Hosp. Psychiat. *2:* 169–176 (1980).

Vincent Mor, PhD, Center for Health Care Research, Brown University, Box G, Providence, RI 02912 (USA)

Adv. psychosom. Med., vol. 18, pp. 135–153 (Karger, Basel 1988)

Cancer's Impact on Caregivers

Andrew E. Slaby

Fair Oaks Hospital, Summit, N.J.; New York University School of Medicine, New York, N.Y.; Brown University, Providence, R.I., USA

Managing patients who are dying, despite our best efforts and all the amenities modern science has wrought, places stress upon caregivers that compromises the sensitivity and humanity required to help the suffering. Patients with advanced cancer and the acquired immune deficiency syndrome (AIDS), require caring when curing is no longer possible. The challenge to the caregiver is enhancement of the quality of life of the moment when promise of future moments is no longer entertained. Pain is mollified, suffering reduced, and social impoverishment managed. Dignity must be preserved as dependence increases and physical being is distorted before patient's and loved ones' own eyes [1]. The physical and emotional vulnerability of those who surround the patient is enhanced as they are confronted with one of the most stressful life events — death of a loved one.

Physicians and nurses generally portrayed as warriors against disease are forced to confront the existential reality of their own limitations as healers as well as the reality that they, their family, their friends, and their lovers may comparably suddenly develop illnesses that result in death even with the finest available medical care. To some this is a challenge. To others, an immense and stressful burden.

Burnout is a common sequela of care of those dying from cancer. Caring turns to apathy; involvement, to distancing. Openness gives way to self-protection as enthusiasm leads to disillusionment and cynicism. Personal devaluation occurs with the erosion of self-esteem concomitant with the helplessness and hopelessness empathetic caregivers experience. Physicians are second only to writers in death from cirrhosis and suffer high rates of drug abuse and suicide [2]. The struggle to come to terms with death has concerned philosophers and theologians from the dawn of history. Today the same questions are asked... and the answers for many, are still wanting.

Stresses Confronting Caregivers

Stresses confronting caregivers vary. It depends on each one's unique constellation of psychological defenses, social supports, previous and current personal losses, philosophy of life, religious ideals, and sensitivity. Life is not being dealt a good hand. It is playing a poor hand well. Each card that is good must be propitiously played to maximize good fortune against a series of bad cards.

Stresses confronting caregivers may be roughly divided into three groups: patient stresses, caregiver stresses, and setting stresses.

Patient Stress

Uncertain Prognosis. The capricious course of many cancers do not allow accurate assessments of expected time course or of expected dates of onset of complications. Patients, families, and caregivers struggle with this uncertainty. Caregivers, like patients' families and friends, may be able to offer only compromised support because of their inability to know how much may be required of them and for how long. Just as a son or daughter may be willing and able to return home for the last week of life of a dying parent *if* they are provided with the hour of death, so too could caregivers more avail themselves if they could calculate the time required to most propitiously extend themselves. Is it days, months, or years? The longer the course of the illness with little response to treatment, the greater the caregiver stress.

Deterioration of the Body and Personality. It is painful to attend the bodily wasting and alteration of personality experienced with tumor growth and spread in some patients, and with oncology treatment (e.g. hair loss, mutilative surgery), in others. Caregivers feel helpless as treatment-resistant cancer takes its course. The deterioration is particularly difficult to confront because what remains intact often reminds the caregiver of better days when the patient was healthy and active. Cancer sometimes leads to organic mental syndromes secondary to decreased oxygen supply to the brain, metabolic changes, metastases, or changes in brain substance. Caregivers, like family members and friends of patients, stand incredulously before individuals who evoke feelings of familiarity but at the same time the individuals appear to be strangers. Patients see themselves in the mirror of the eyes of those who behold them as well as in actual mirrors. Both mirrors serve to enhance anxiety of the patient as the eyes of those who attend them convey to the patient's progress of disease. The anxiety and fear of the patient is felt by empathetic caregivers who are aware of the communication to patients by what they look at and what they do not and by how much or how little time they spend with a patient.

Withdrawal. During the process of dying, there is a natural tendency for the person dying and for those around him or her to withdraw. This is a protective response. Loss is inevitable. One must begin to invest in others. For patients there may be excessive concern with their own needs and anger that they cannot be met, particularly the need to be saved and live. Family and caregivers find themselves turning to those who will survive and who are their future, not to those who will soon be history. The continued requirement of caregivers for interaction with dying patients in a responsive and responsible way taxes this adaptive response [3–7]. Caregivers, unlike patients and family, cannot withdraw to protect themselves from the impact of continued confrontation with pain and loss.

Nature of Death. Particulars of an individual death enhance or diminish stress. Long suffering, intractable pain, disfigurement, and loss of dignity through delirium and bowel or urinary incontinence, or death by suicide enhance it. Sudden and painless or minimally painful death are easier to accept. Thomas Browne, who authored *Religio Medici* in 1643, cautioned that most who pass through life take health for granted but Browne, a pathologist, who knew the thousand doors to death, thanked God that he could die but once. So too, do caregivers who have experienced the many faces of death by cancer. While more than half of individuals who have cancer die from other causes, those who do die consume considerable medical and psychological resources, testing and draining caregivers, families, and friends.

Dependency. Patients with cancer and their families are more dependent on caregivers than patients with other illnesses. Patients with cardiac disease exercise, meditate, lose weight, change their diet and take medication to contribute personally to increasing risk of survival. Much of the therapy of cancer patients requires medical assistance: intravenous chemotherapy, radiation and surgery. Diet and exercise have little impact. Greater dependency on physicians and nurses humiliates many patients and taxes caregivers. Dependency varies with number of supportive family members and friends available but always is present to some degree. This dependency and the resentment associated with it that is felt by patients particularly when they, if they were previously quite independent as many professional and business men and women are, engenders the same feelings in caregivers that parents feel faced with many dependent children who resent having to ask for what they want and plan their lives around their parents', rather than their own time needs.

Patients' and Families' Anger. Frustration leads to anger. Frustrated families get angry with caregivers. Frustrated caregivers, at patients' families. Frustrated patients, at both. Why wasn't help sought earlier? Why didn't a doctor recognize a warning sign? Why isn't a nurse or doctor more attentive? Why can't something be done to alleviate the pain? All these questions are valid. All can be asked. All, however, do not have simple answers. Most symptoms people have are without consequence. When malignancy is discovered, suddenly everything retrospectively becomes apparent. If nothing had happened, no more would have been made of a symptom. Marcel Proust once said, when all is copecetic we do not attend to nuances. Persons in pain, in contrast, listen to their body like lovers to the words of their beloved. Those around patients do not share pain to the same degree and therefore do not attend to the same degree.

Repeated Personal Loss. Caregivers are human beings. We all have histories. Our unique personal pasts color all we see and do. In many instances, past personal tragedy is a motivating factor in occupational choice. Early, recent and impending losses work synergistically to enhance caregivers' sensitivity to deaths of patients. They feel new pain, grief and helplessness. Often the desire to provide care for those in need is predicated on a wish to do for others as we would have liked to have done for others in our past and pray be done for ourselves when need arises. This is called altruism and, as such, is a healthy defense against feelings of helplessness to care for others we experienced in the past. We care for others as we ourselves want to be cared for. Sometimes, it is not sufficient. We feel too much of the past and the present is too present. There are limits to pain even the most psychologically resourceful of us can experience. If one sees in repeated dying patients, a lost mother, father, sibling, spouse, lover or child, grief is rewakened and experienced anew. If our own need to be cared for ourselves in a way we would like is not fulfilled, we feel empty and even more needy, given the drain on our own resources. To care well, we must also be cared for well.

Caregiver Factors

Role Ambiguity. Teams mollify stress as stress is shared and dispersed. Lack of clear definition of role on a team, however, enhances stress and incites anger when burden of care shifts unexpectedly or is disproportionately allocated. Teams evolve slowly and painfully. The process is continuous [2]. Absence of clear job descriptions militates against coordinated care and enhances stress.

Economic Burden. Human resources, social and economic, are limited. We wish we could give all to patients and to those who care for our patients. Medical care, like education, is a human right not a privilege. Both should be provided for all wishing and requiring it. The cost of a debilitating illness such as cancer is a threat to the immediate security of a patient and to the long-term security of the family. Caregivers want to deliver the highest quality of care. Understaffing and absence of critical team members stresses caregivers and patients alike [8]. Compromises made because of limited economic or psychological resources may be necessary and understandable but are never easy. Psychosocial aspects of care are the first to be sacrificed in hard times by hospitals and diminished in value by third-party payers. Ironically, in cancer more than most other illnesses, psychosocial support for a significant component of the course of illness may be the most important element in patient management.

The Idea of Death. The idea that we all *must* die haunts many like no other human experience. The fear may be unconsciously denied or not discussed but is omnipresent. Children and religion offer immortality to some. Money and power, temporary control. All these however give way, save for a few with intense religious faith, when an individual is repeatedly confronted with the reality of death oncological caregivers must experience daily. Those who care for cancer patients must either directly confront their own mortality or expend psychic energy to mollify the intensity of the reality to allow for some reconciliation with the idea of death. There is an ironic benefit of this daily confrontation. Plato enjoined us to contemplate death, to live life. The cost of denial for some is that so much effort is expended in denying that too soon they are old and, too quickly, dead. Confrontation of death dictates life be lived more fully, and each second of good fortune savored like a ripe strawberry dipped in champagne begging to be devoured and wanting to please.

Caregiver Anger. Caregivers experience anger [4, 9] when patients refuse treatment, when they appear for treatment too late, when patients do not do well, when they cannot cure patients, and when excessive demands are placed upon them by patients, families and other caregivers. Overidentification with patients and their helplessness leads to personal devaluation. Why can't I do better? Why can't I relieve the pain? Why can't I control side effects? Or the obverse from patients and families: Why can't you (read caregivers) do better? Why can't *you* relieve the pain? Why can't *you* control side effects? These demands are understandable but in many instances unreasonable given the state of oncology. Understanding does not assuage feeling. Anger is a natural response to demands that are humanly impossible to fulfill no matter how much we wish we could. Anger drains. Sustained anger contributes to burnout.

Burnout. Attrition in oncology tends to occur early, either from burnout or from dislike of the work [4] or after many years of service without reprieve. Burnout is *both* a result of stress and a stressor. It is a stressor to those experiencing it impacting on how they respond to colleagues, family and friends, and to the colleagues, family and friends confronted with a burnout person. Burnout occurs in any profession or social situation when excessive demands are placed on individuals' energy, strength and resources. In such instances, individuals wear out and become exhausted. They lose enthusiasm, become depressed, and doubt ability to heal and lead. They become cynical, disillusioned and angry. They dread going to work. Headache, diarrhea, indigestion and sleep disturbance are frequent. It is common among nurses and physicians treating large numbers of patients who die. To counter burnout and the effects of burnout in all we do and in all we encounter requires a concerted effort to reduce stress in every way possible. The preservation of enthusiasm and sensitivity requires an active program of stress reduction by caregivers.

Role Conflict. Medical professionals are mandated to fight disease to help people live. It has not been their mission for decades to help people die peacably. Caring enough to help people die with dignity, even if it shortens their lives, is an ironic paradox. Even more difficult is the need to change roles in the course of management of a patient with cancer who has a recurrence that is not treatable, from that of a healer to that of a facilitator (literally one who makes dying easier). Since most people do not die of cancer when it occurs, the change in set can come quite unexpectedly as it does with a woman free of cancer of the breast for 17 years and considered cured, whose physician discovers metastases and she goes on to die of it. Helping people live and helping people die peacably and with dignity is not a conflict if a caregiver defines his or her task as caring in addition to curing. When curing is no longer possible, then caring becomes the primary task. Hospitals were founded centuries ago to care before curing was possible.

Fear of Criticism. Retrospective analysis of a situation is more comfortable than bearing responsibility for decisions at the time of an event. Managing cancer patients is probably the most difficult medical task. Fear of making a wrong and fatal choice is why so many patients wish to defer treatment decisions to physicians or a care team who presumably operates from a greater experiental and knowledge base. If a woman elects a lumpectomy rather than a mastectomy and goes on to die, the burden of personal choice is on her shoulders. If, however, a physician or care team suggested the latter and it proves by outcome to have been an incorrect choice or is assumed to be (metastases could have occurred prior to mastectomy), the caregivers are seen as responsible. The worst regrets are what may have been. Caregivers assuming responsibility for choices will relieve the self-abnegation of a dying patient but enhance that of a caregiver. AIDS currently does not have a potential cure at present and therefore early diagnosis and treatment choice do not play a critical role to patient or caregiver as does the reality of just having a disease of which 100% at the present time die.

Technical Stress. The field of oncology is rapidly changing. What was fatal two decades ago such as Hodgkin's disease is now a therapeutic challenge with a remarkable cure rate. Techniques of pain management and of treatment of delirium comparably are advancing at such a rate that caregivers recently trained are more aware of state-of-the-art care than those who are not in academic centers and continually involved in continuing medical educational activities. Requirements for continuing medical education are greater than earlier in this century when caring rather than curing was the mission of hospitals. Today there exists continued stress to remain state-of-the-art while at the same time maintaining continuity of care and availability to patients and other members of the caregiving team.

Lack of Preparation for Tasks Associated with Management of Oncology Patients. The great thrust of training in most health science centers is on the technical aspects of health care. Caregivers managing cancer patients are confronted with tasks requiring understanding of both patients and their own psychodynamics and of how past experience with helplessness and care providers determines response to the current situation. In addition, they must understand how systems function to facilitate good care in the hospitals and obtain support and compliance with treatment from family systems. Staff must learn to manage people and relationships whose behavior will impact on patients' mood and course as well as on their own mood and ability to treat [1, 10, 11]. Lack of preparation for these tasks leaves much to the caprice of experience and encounters with individuals who help conceptualize tasks in a language that facilitates understanding and behavior modification to enhance better care.

Pressure to Cure. Denial of extent or phase of illness and limits of care leads to ill-advised persistence in therapeutic efforts, medically and surgically, beyond what is clinically indicated [1]. The cost is further discomfort for a patient, a waste of limited medical resources, and further caregiver stress.

Fatigue. Exhausted and overworked nurses and physicians cannot provide optimal care. It is impossible to care anymore than love if we are not cared for or loved ourselves. We are not endless wellsprings of succor and sustenance.

Inability to Share Feelings. Caregivers suffer and, hopefully, enjoy the same spectrum of emotion patients do. After all, one day a person may be a caregiver and the next day be a patient. This is a factor in the stress of caregiving. There are, however, few legitimate vehicles for ventilation. Feelings get pent up. Ethics of confidentiality and professional etiquette dictate ad hominum feelings be sparingly discharged — in many instances only to a therapist or clergyman. Words unspoken can lead to emotional abscesses which, if unlanced, erode at our being or explode into marital and family discord.

Desire to Provide Holistic Care. Doctors and nurses are charged with holistic care. Outcome is to be wholeness. All needs of patients are to be addressed, not just abstract laboratory values [12, 13]. Nurses even more than doctors are expected to be coordinators, family therapists, assessors, medical providers, and delineators of needs. The demands of some oncology patients require a dimension of attentiveness few care systems can provide. A personal relationship between a doctor or nurse and a patient is the best way to provide care. This is the underlying philosophy of primary care medicine and nursing. Primary caregivers must take assaults, anger, withdrawal and negativism without acting in kind. This may be effected in the short run. In the long run, however, this results in development of automatons, the worst caricature of medicine in the technologic era. Only robots do not feel and respond.

Guilt. Caregivers, perhaps more than most others, experience guilt. They feel badly if they do not provide the best of care... and they should... if they aspire to the best. But, they are not God. Technical mistakes occur. A caregiver may have minimized the importance of pain that ultimately heralded the onset of metastases. At these times, and others, caregivers may have done all that is humanly possible. Still, patients go on to die. Tolerating the guilt that makes one successful and good but also troubled when inevitable tragedies occur over which one has no control is one of the most difficult adult tasks. The ability to tolerate irrational guilt is not enhanced when bereft family and friends, frightened patients, or guilty caregivers attempt to allocate guilt on the most sensitive of those who care.

Setting Factors

Atmosphere of Care Facility. Environments serve to mollify and intensify stress. Crowded, noisy facilities without privacy tax caregivers' efforts to maintain patient dignity and focus their own efforts. Hospitals, as opposed to hospices and home care, can be particularly alienating environments. The atmosphere of the care setting is one of the most simple factors contributing to patient and caregivers' stress to reduce, yet, ironically, short-sighted hospital administrators fail to provide a setting which will reduce staff attrition and make patients and their families more comfortable.

Technical Emphasis of Modern Oncology. Contemporary oncology is highly technologically oriented. Patients are often placed in protocols that some research-oriented and many nonresearch-oriented clinicians find impersonal. These protocols work in many cases but also are attended by many side effects including hair loss, diarrhea, and nausea. The lack of immediate results and uncertainty of long-term cure frustrates and compounds the stress of caregivers who are themselves conflicted over treatment programs when confronted by families' and patients' concerns over the issues they themselves struggle with daily.

Absence of Clinical Role Models. We all need mentors. Learning does not occur in a vacuum. We look to others for answers to that which we currently cannot or have not yet learned to provide. The absence of such means we must learn by the painful process of experience. This is time-consuming and draining. Role models facilitate new learning and reinforce old.

Time Constraints. It is impossible for a sentient person to ask if someone is alone, in pain, or wishes to talk and then not address the issue. Yet, caregivers are consumed by ever changing demands, some of urgent need. Feeling caregivers are in a double-bind caught between the devil and the deep blue sea. If they ask how a person feels and then cut them off to attend to another patient, they experience the disappointment of patients. If they don't ask, they know they do not practice holistic care. Caregiving like parenthood is sometimes a no-win situation.

Managing Caregiver Stress

Successful management of caregiver stress entails understanding systems. Caregivers do not exist in a vacuum anymore than patients do. Their surroundings enhance or reduce stress. Staff-staff, staff-patient, staff-family, and staff-friend interactions must be understood to mollify stress and maximize quality of care provided through support of caregivers. It is often simplistically put that to love another you must first be able to love yourself. Caregivers, as mentioned earlier, cannot care if they do not first care for themselves and are cared for. Caregiving systems which most effectively provide holistic oncological care are designed to promote caregiver growth, enhance caregiver bonding, counter burnout, and respect the person of *both* patient and caregiver. Reducing caregiver stress requires reducing factors in patients and caregivers' lives and in the setting that contributes to stress so that inevitable tensions that emerge not only are tolerable but contribute actively to enhancing quality of care provided.

Patient Factors

Hope. The ancient Greeks felt the most tragic of ills was not dying but dying alone. Hope is needed to live each moment of life fully, even the last. Hope is essential to validate the efforts of a caregiver. Most individuals who suffer cancer *do not* succumb to it. Cancer in its late stages is serious but never without hope. Miracle recoveries, albeit rare, are reported. Those much healthier may predecease someone ill. The quality of extant being is more a measure of success of treatment than prolonged physiologic functioning. Many people outlive physiologically, well-being psychologically. Hope is essential to patients and critical to counteract burnout and to enhance esprit de corps of a team.

Limit Settings. Effective functioning is sustained only if limits of personal giving are established [2]. No one can totally fulfill the needs of another, much less a patient with a family, all of whom have rapidly changing needs given the realities of cancer and its treatment . Individuals on a team are still individuals. They need privacy and time to refresh themselves. If any one member of a team provides their home telephone number to a patient or a family, he/she will disproportionately experience the burden of care. An on-call schedule is necessary so that all team members share in both providing care for patients and for themselves, Firm limit setting is the first step in assuring quality of care. We all must know what we can reasonably do and what is beyond our limit to reasonably provide.

Family Support. At first glance, emphasis on family support seems more for patients than caregiver benefit. In fact, however, the more families concur with treatment plans and are aware of illness course and the risks and benefits of treatment, the less staff will be the object of displaced anger from family members who, like patients, feel helpless. Developing relationships with family through individual family meetings, family groups, support groups and educational activities facilitates staff functioning by reduction in displaced hostility and in the number of telephone calls and requests for meetings when anticipated but undesirable effects of illness and treatment occur.

Psychiatric Consultation. Psychiatric consultation individually or in groups on a weekly basis provides an opportunity for staff to learn how to help patients cope with feelings as well as for staff themselves to learn to cope with their own and other caregivers' feelings [4]. When done in a group setting, this fosters development of bonding and trust as ways of helping patients and caregivers themselves are elaborated and implemented.

Dignity. This often overlooked factor is one that has considerable implication in reduction of stress of patients, family and staff. When patients feel vulnerable to the caprice of cancer and staff to the caprice of their patients' and own emotions, a self-conscious effort to treat patients, other staff, and family with dignity, goes a long way in supporting satisfactory functioning and in helping patients feel in control of stress [1]. Life is not being dealt a good hand, but playing a poor hand well. If you treat others with respect and dignity, you engender respect and treatment with dignity yourself. Addressing patients formally until a relationship evolves that merits greater familiarity makes patients feel that just because they are seriously ill, they are not less of persons. They are still *persons to be respected.* In this way, caregivers themselves are seen as people to be respected in a collaborative search for answers to illness and not objects of anxiety or fear. Two people with dignity can respect each other as well as their own limitations. This reduces stress of the anger from vulnerable patients who feel 'one down' as well as the stress of unrealistic expectations.

Caregiver Factors

Accepting Patients as They Are. It is difficult to change adult defenses under the best of circumstances. It is all the more so when all extant defenses are called upon to handle the crisis of life-threatening illness. It is a difficult enough task to help a patient accept the reality of cancer and its treatment. We do not have to add to the stress by trying to make patients accept a disease as we think they should rather than in the way that is right for them as they are. The first step in accepting patients as they are is accepting ourselves as we are. Both reduce stress by accepting reality and learning to cope with it as it is, not as what we wish it to be. This acceptance has the same salving effect as the absent witness exercise described by Weissman [6].

Stress Awareness. Stress is inevitable. No matter how hard we try, we will experience it. Stress itself, however, does not destroy. Bertrand Russell taught us that it is not the experience that happens to us, but what we do with experience that happens to us. To manage stress and care for our patients, ourselves, and other caregivers we must first identify stress in ourselves and in others [2]. This allows means of dissipating it or using it for creative growth. One creative use of experiencing the stress of daily contact with cancer is to use the experience to live more fully ourselves and derive greater richness from each moment we experience alone and together with someone we love [4].

Support Groups. Pain bonds individuals more than pleasure. Suicide rates fall in times of war and rise in times of prosperity. We need others at times of strife. Treating patients, some of whom are terminally ill, and others who may be in the relatively near future is a time of strife. This is coupled, of course, with the constant presence of discomforting effects of treatment even when successful. The ambiguity of prognosis and the ravages of oncotherapy is common to nearly all. All those who are in professional caring roles know this stress more than spouses, lovers, children, parents, friends and colleagues in other areas. Therefore the most natural and appropriate support group is one composed solely of those treating patients with cancer [14]. Those who experience the parameters of the stress can support each other as they ventilate and seek ways to cope with caring. Support groups serve not only to explore and recognize anxieties and stress produced in the caregiver as a result of working with oncology patients, but also to assist staff in developing and implementing therapeutic responses to psychological issues of the patients in evaluating and treating patients with psychological issues surrounding their illness, and in developing and implementing psychological research projects [15].

Individual Coping Styles. No two individuals use the same constellation of defenses to adapt to stresses of caring for cancer patients. Some deny the threat to life experienced by their patients. Others cope by seeing pain and suffering as part of a scheme whereby God helps us become better through suffering. Strong religious faith facilitates adaptation to the stresses of seeing people suffer and die by conceptualizing human woe as part of a process for which there is eternal reward. It is the belief in some religions that we die into Eternal Life. Unfortunately, not all of us have such faith and, even if we do, it falters at times. Others employ humor to cope with the stresses of caregiving while still others try to control that which they can to compensate for anxiety and depression suffered from not controlling other aspects. For a team to function effectively, members must know and respect each other's coping styles. Some styles are destructive, however, and cannot be tolerated. If a caregiver must deny the significance of a symptom heralding a recurrence, palliative treatment may be foregone. Comparably, controlling others to assuage one's lack of control over cancer or its treatment is destructive to team spirit and to patients.

Psychotherapy. Conflicts from early life, long laid dormant, may reemerge as one treats an individual with an illness over which there is little control [16]. Anger, frustration, anxiety and grief from unresolved personal experiences in the past reemerge in the face of a life-threatening illness [17]. All contemporary human experience is interpreted in terms of past experience. The meaning of cancer and its management are different for each caregiver. How one has managed previous crises and manages current ones is determined by intelligence, affectional endowment, vocational and educational achievement, and early and more recent life experiences. Unless one has grown through previous crises, individuals with previous psychosocial difficulties have been found to be more likely to feel worthless, unattractive, embittered, victimized, and depressed when seeing the impact of cancer and its treatment on patients and their families. This may be especially true if someone close to the caregiver resembles the patient and suffers the same fate. In such instances, personal psychotherapy may be required to help integrate the past experience and resolve still lingering conflicts to improve functioning and reduce stress.

Leisure Activity. Leisure activities are important in caregiver stress reduction. If off-work hours are consumed by domestic drudgery and childrearing, the absence of time to one's self to reflect and relax serves to enhance rather than reduce work stress. Most activities that are relaxing have in common a change in set sometimes to the extent that the mind is on vacation. Some jog or exercise in other ways. Others listen to music, paint, sew, cook, meditate, read or simply walk or sit and be with one's self.

Empathetic Friends. Caring is draining but obviously rewarding on a fundamental level or we would not do it. Because it is draining and because we are aware of the tax on ourselves, we listen for appreciation from those we care for and their significant others as well as from our own friends and family. We want them to know our days are not always easy. We may not always be as available to listen and serve friends when we are all listened out and tired. We may want to make love... or at times want to but can't because of preoccupation with others' woes, with life's unfairness. Our hearts can want but our bodies have been numbed. We must tune down to tune into our own and others', who are not our patients, needs. George Eliot wrote in her book, *Daniel Deronda*, that the greatest principle of growth lies in human choice. Who we choose to surround ourselves with determines how we will feel about who we are and what we do. Friends enhance or diminish self-esteem. They support... or undercut. They create safe landings to mollify our failing at certain risks... or forever discourage our desire to be. Those who care for patients with a potentially devastating illness, an illness in which their own cells are devouring them from within, need good empathetic friends who intuit the pain and stress even if they themselves have not had the same experience. Nothing helps one to understand as much as to be understood.

Absent Witness. Weissman [6] describes a procedure whereby guilt over what one has not done is reduced and thereby stress reduced, referred to as the *absent witness* exercise. This can involve one or a group of caregivers. In the exercise, a former patient, perhaps one who has died, is called up in fantasy to query what more could have been done. What did they want short of full recovery that they did not get? Through this process, demoralized caregivers more easily come to distinguish between 'should' and 'could' and between guilt and undue expectations. Man proposes, God disposes. It is not always humanly possible to provide what demoralized guilty teams believe is due. If the caregiver were the patient, what more could he/she have reasonably expected. The reason so many people avoided care of cancer patients until recently was the absence of ability to provide cure or palliation in a sufficient number of instances. The prize to the caregiver team who has undertaken the absent witness exercise is awareness that they usually have done all that which is humanly possible. Over time the caregivers come to realize that the criteria of success is that they are state-of-the-art, not that they are God. The absent witness procedure is essentially an exercise in reality testing employed to convince caregivers that feelings of worthlessness and despair are irrational so that they may function more effectively [4].

Goal Clarification. Stress occurs when uncertainty exists as to where we are going or what we are striving for. Delineation of a goal, for instance caring rather than curing in a hospice situation, reduces confusion and stress by reducing a need to hope to cure the patients. Pain management and psychosocial support assume priority over future attempts to arrest disease [18].

Setting Factors

Environment. Our physical surroundings as well as the people we work with determine how we feel about what we are doing and contribute to our evolving identity as a person and a caregiver. A selection of people for a team who share a desire to provide the best, not just very good, care and a sensitivity to patient as person, enhances bonding among members and reduction of stress. A physical environment that is designed to protect privacy, provide comfort, and evince a respect for a person at his/her most vulnerable moment acts synergistically with caregiver characteristics to attenuate stress and enhance self-esteem of both caregiver and patient.

Team Organization. Responsibility commensurate with level of training and acquired skill enhances productivity and reduces stress [2]. Mechanisms should be built into the team to review its organization, communication among members, and how it manages conflict to maximize functioning and minimize stress.

Working Conditions. Stress is reduced through assuring stability in scheduling and expected activities. Patient and staff emergencies may arise leading to a temporary heightening of stress due to greater workload or changed hours but this should be an exception, not a rule. Regular hours, defined tasks, clear lines of accountability, and allocation of responsibility by skill and training, reduces stress and increases morale. When sudden changes in working hours are dictated by staff illness or unexpected attrition, additional sleep, decreased food and drink intake, and arrangement of most important activities during peak hours reduces stress [2].

Interdisciplinary Effort. All health professionals share the same goal: to care and to cure where possible. Each caregiver's unique expertise, however, is varied by training and professional experience [19]. Social workers mobilize community resources. Psychologists evaluate neuropsychological functioning, provide psychotherapy, and reduce pain by behavioral interventions. Nurses monitor course of illness and response to treatment and treatment side effects. Clergy attend to the spiritual needs of patients, family and staff. Physicians specifically trained in oncology bring to bear state-of-art chemotherapy, radiotherapy and surgery. Calling upon each individual to provide what they do know best results in the highest quality of care a team as a whole can provide. When tasks are assumed by those without proper qualifications due to limited staffing and poorly defined responsibility stress is increased and those without the best knowledge are called upon to do what others on the team could do better and more efficiently. Psychiatrists complete the constellation of expertise on a team with their special awareness of how patients' and staffs' behavior is determined by the complex interplay of biological, social, psychological and existential forces.

Continuing Education. Infrequently included among those things that assuage stress is continuing education. This is another example of being cared for so you can care better. It is also a factor that increases morale by enhancing the self-esteem of the caregiver. If a caregiver is state-of-the-art, and maintaining that state is seen as an institutional priority, the caregiver feels special and is perceived as such by others.

Research. This, like continuing education, helps keep caregivers state-of-the-art if the research is at the cutting edge as well as enhance self-esteem by the perception of patients and community that a particular oncology group is seen as special. It adds a third factor that is unique to itself. Research efforts provide hope. A cure may not be here today but researchers are working on it before patients' eyes. They may yet benefit from it themselves.

Collaboration. Varied input and varying opportunities for support make the task of caregivers easier. It is impossible to do everything ourselves. Recognizing this fact is not only a sign of maturity, it is a major factor in stress reduction. The most cost-effective way to share the burden is the use of trained, supervised volunteers in gathering data, patient education and providing family and patient support [2]. Creative use of other hospital personnel, such as nutritionists, psychologists, social workers, psychiatrists, clergy, music therapists, creative therapists, occupational therapists and physical therapists on a regular basis, provides an atmosphere of caring and sharing the burden of task. Caregivers feel the load less individually, thus lightening the burden of care while strengthening esprit de corps by having the higher quality program that such a mosaic of talent provides.

Support Teams. Support teams are groups of people who gather to ventilate and share feelings. They allow expression of anger toward patients and other staff as well as of guilt, frustration, despair and professional malaise. To best provide a vehicle for emotional expression, teams should be composed of naturally companionable groups. If nurses feel freer to ventilate with other nurses and physicians with other physicians, groups are composed along disciplinary lines. With well-functioning teams, the team itself may become the nucleus of the group. Facilitators of such groups include clergy, psychiatrists, psychologists, psychiatric nurses, and psychiatric social workers.

Conclusions

Nowhere is the task for caregivers as well as for patients' families and patients as awesome as with cancer and cancer-like illnesses, such as AIDS, which are incompletely understood and often fatal. The challenge to the caregiver is to maintain sensitivity and technical skill while at the same time not be overwhelmed with the pain of empathy and with the fatigue of caring and curing. It is not an impossible challenge, but indeed a Promethian one. It is made easier and less stressful when the caregivers accept themselves as human beings and, after that, learn acceptance of self and their patients.

Caregivers have limits. They are not inexhaustible fonts of emotional sensitivity nor, for that matter, are they physically indefatigable. They have needs to be fulfilled and lives that go beyond their professional activities. Setting limits and sharing tasks in a team reduces the burden. Ventilation in support groups and the salve of friends and colleagues sharing mollifies the stress and provides a supportive framework for growth in the face of one of humankind's oldest adversaries, cancer.

References

1 Gonda, T.A.; Ruark, J.E.: Dying dignified: the health professionals guide to care (Addison-Wesley, London 1984).
2 Mount, B.M.: Dealing with our losses. J. clin. Oncol. *4:* 1127–1134 (1986).
3 Renneker, R.E.: Countertransference reactions to cancer. Psychosom. Med. *19:* 409–418 (1957).
4 Slaby, A.E.; Glicksman, A.S.: Adapting to life-threatening illness (Praeger Press, New York 1985).
5 Wahl, C.W.: The physician's treatment of the dying patient. Ann. N.Y. Acad. Sci. *164:* 759–775 (1969).
6 Weissman, A.D.: Understanding the cancer patient: the syndrome of caregiver's plight. Psychiatry *44:* 161–168 (1981).
7 White, L.P.: The self-image of the physician and the care of dying patients. Ann. N.Y. Acad. Sci. *164:* 822–831 (1969).
8 Kocher, G.P.: Coping with a death from cancer. J. consult. clin. Psychol. *54:* 623–631 (1986).

9 Cassem, N.H.: The dying patient; in Hackett, Cassem, MGH handbook of general hospital psychiatry, pp. 300–318 (Mosby, St Louis 1978).
10 Strauss, A.: Family and staff during last weeks and days of terminal illness. Ann. N.Y. Acad. Sci. *164:* 687–693 (1969).
11 Prichard, R.: Dying — some issues and problems. Ann. N.Y. Acad. Sci. *162:* 707–717 (1967).
12 Roberts, S.L.: The critical care nurse as an open system; in Roberts, Behavioral concepts and the critically ill patient, pp. 335–351 (Prentice-Hall, Englewood Cliffs 1976).
13 Roberts, S.L.: Behavioral concepts and the critically ill patient (Prentice-Hall, Englewood Cliffs 1976).
14 Taerk, G.: Psychological support of oncology nurses: a role for the liaison psychiatrist. Can. J. Psychiat. *28:* 532–535 (1983).
15 Tull, R.; Glicksman, A.S.; Hilderlay, L.; Tefft, M.: Psychosocial support in an oncology facility. Proc. AACR and ASCO, p. 394 (1981).
16 Needleman, J.: The perception of mortality. Ann. N.Y. Acad. Sci. *164:* 733–738 (1969).
17 Garfield, C.A.: Elements of psychosocial oncology: doctor-patient relationships in terminal illness; in Garfield, Psychosocial care of the dying patient, pp. 102–118 (McGraw-Hill, New York 1978).
18 Strain, J.J.; Grossman, S.: Psychological care of the medically ill: a primer in liaison psychiatry, pp. 138–148 (ACC, East Norwalk 1975).
19 Hartl, D.E.: Stress management and the nurse; in Sutterley, Donnelly, Stress management (Aspen Systems, Germantown 1979).

Andrew E. Slaby, MD, PhD, MPH, Fair Oaks Hospital,
Summit, NJ 07901 (USA)

Subject Index